WE170 HAM

is book is to be returned on or before
the last date stamped below.

25. JUL 1996

LIMB AMPUTATION

FORTHCOMING TITLES

Occupational Therapy for the Brain-Injured Adult
Jo Clark-Wilson and Gordon Muir Giles

Modern Electrotherapy
Mary Dyson and Christopher Hayne

Physiotherapy in Respiratory Care
Alexandra Hough

Speech and Language Problems in Children
Dilys A. Treharne

THERAPY IN PRACTICE SERIES

Edited by Jo Campling

This series of books is aimed at 'therapists' concerned with rehabilitation in a very broad sense. The intended audience particularly includes occupational therapists, physiotherapists and speech therapists, but many titles will also be of interest to nurses, psychologists, medical staff, social workers, teachers or volunteer workers. Some volumes are interdisciplinary, others are aimed at one particular profession. All titles will be comprehensive but concise, and practical but with due reference to relevant theory and evidence. They are not research monographs but focus on professional practice, and will be of value to both students and qualified personnel.

1. Occupational Therapy for Children with Disabilities
   Dorothy E. Penso
2. Living Skills for Mentally Handicapped People
   Christine Peck and Chia Swee Hong
3. Rehabilitation of the Older Patient
   Edited by Amanda J. Squires
4. Physiotherapy and the Elderly Patient
   Paul Wagstaff and Davis Coakley
5. Rehabilitation of the Severely Brain-Injured Adult
   Edited by Ian Fussey and Gordon Muir Giles
6. Communication Problems in Elderly People
   Rosemary Gravell
7. Occupational Therapy Practice in Psychiatry
   Linda Finlay
8. Working with Bilingual Language Disability
   Edited by Deirdre M. Duncan
9. Counselling Skills for Health Professionals
   Philip Burnard
10. Teaching Interpersonal Skills
    A handbook of experiential learning for health professionals
    Philip Burnard
11. Occupational Therapy for Stroke Rehabilitation
    Simon Thompson and Maryanne Morgan
12. Assessing Physically Disabled People at Home
    Kathy Maczka

Limb Amputation
From aetiology to rehabilitation

R. Ham and L. Cotton

Therapy in Practice 23

CHAPMAN & HALL

London · New York · Tokyo · Melbourne · Madras

UK   Chapman and Hall, 2–6 Boundary Row, London SE1 8HN
USA   Chapman and Hall, 29 West 35th Street, New York NY10001
JAPAN   Chapman and Hall Japan, Thomson Publishing Japan, Hirakawacho
            Nemoto Building, 7F, 1–7–11 Hirakawa-cho, Chiyoda-ku, Tokyo 102
AUSTRALIA   Chapman and Hall Australia, Thomas Nelson Australia, 102 Dodds
            Street, South Melbourne, Victoria 3205
INDIA   Chapman and Hall India, R. Seshadri, 32 Second Main Road, CIT East,
            Madras 600 035

First edition 1991

© 1991 R. Ham and L. Cotton

Typeset in 10/12pt Times by Best-set Typesetter Ltd
Printed in Great Britain by St Edmundsbury Press Ltd,
Bury St Edmunds, Suffolk

ISBN 0 412 34610 9

British Library Cataloguing in Publication Data
Cotton, L.
    Limb amputation.
    1. Man. Limbs. Amputation
    I. Title II. Ham, R. III. Series
    617.58059
ISBN 0 412 34610 9

Library of Congress Cataloging-in-Publication Data
Cotton, L.T. (Leonard T.)
    Limb amputation: from aetiology to rehabilitation / L. Cotton and
    R. Ham — 1st ed.
        p.   cm. — (Therapy in practice series; 23)
    Includes bibliographical references.
    Includes index.
    ISBN 0-412-34610-9
    1. Amputation. 2. Amputations of leg. 3. Amputees —
Rehabilitation. I. Ham, R. (Rosalind), 1952–   . II. Title.
III. Series.
    [DNLM: 1. Amputation—methods. 2. Amputees—psychology.
3. Amputees—rehabilitation 4. Artificial Limbs—rehabilitation.
WE 170 C851L]
RD553.C68   1991
617.5'8059—dc20
DNLM/DLC
for Library of Congress   90-15063
                                                               CIP

Contents

Acknowledgements

We would first like to acknowledge Lindis Richards and June de Trafford, both members of this department, without whose typing, computing, late evening and weekend support this book could not have been finished. Our thanks and acknowledgement also go to members of the hospital team and colleagues who gave us information and their valuable time by reading the appropriate scripts, especially David Thornberry, Pam Barsby, Kathy Leason, Sue Douglas and Kathy O'Kelly.

We would also like to thank Professor Colin Roberts, Professor of Medical Engineering and Medical Physics, for his support and use of his department's equipment during the preparation of this book.

We acknowledge and are grateful to Setons, Remploy, LIC, Vessa Ltd and Blatchfords Ltd and thank them for allowing us to reproduce their material.

Finally we would like to thank our spouses for their constant support and·excellent culinary skills during the writing and preparation of this book.

R. Ham
L.T. Cotton
May 1990

Preface

The majority of amputations in the western world today are due to vascular disease. Despite the advances in surgical treatment of this disease, particularly by reconstruction, it is a sad fact that the number of amputations performed in these countries each year for vascular disease is increasing.

Most of these amputees are elderly and their life expectancy is short, so it is important that the treatment and rehabilitation that they receive is informed, appropriate, efficient and swift to enable them to return successfully to life in the community for their remaining years.

Management of this group of patients has proved to be successful only if a multidisciplinary team approach is adopted. Until recently in the UK, this approach sadly has only been implemented by a few centres. However, with the publication of the McColl report into the prosthetic and wheelchair service in 1986, interest in the care of the amputee is growing throughout the country.

This book covers all aspects of amputation from disease and diagnosis to rehabilitation and community discharge with emphasis on the management of the largest group, the vascular lower limb amputee. A team approach is described and emphasized as being essential for good results and subsequent successful return into the community. The role of each of the important disciplines is described in relation to the appropriate part of the rehabilitation phase.

This book is intended for all staff who are dealing with amputees, to give them knowledge of the best methods of management and good practice.

1

The history of amputation surgery and prosthetics

AMPUTATION SURGERY

The word amputation derives from the Latin *amputare*, which means cutting around.

Early history

Amputated limbs were found in the remains of Neolithic man from the late Stone Age, approximately 2000 BC, but the reasons for the amputations can only be speculated (Isherwood, 1980). It is thought that they are most likely to have been due to trauma or punishment and not for disease or surgical reasons. Both in the Old Testament and in the Egyptian medical writings there is no mention of surgical amputation but recent examination of Egyptian mummies has shown the presence of arterial disease (Ruffer, 1921). The majority of these amputations appear to have been due to trauma or congenital limb loss and the prostheses were placed in tombs by the embalmers, it is thought, purely for reincarnation purposes as there is no record of their being used in life (Butler, 1986).

The Greek physician, Hippocrates of Cos (460–380 BC) in his essays or treatise *On Joints*, wrote the first description of amputation for vascular gangrene. He described removal of the blackened tissue at the joint above the area of demarcation and autoamputation. At this time Greek medicine was advanced and the Greek surgeon of the day was familiar with the tourniquet, surgical drains, cautery, surgical cleanliness and the use of wine and vinegar as methods of antisepsis (Isherwood, 1980).

Celsus, a Roman in the first century AD, recommended amputation between healthy and gangrenous tissue 'best some healthy tissue be removed rather than leave any diseased tissue'. He also described ligation of the bleeding vessels, division of the bone at a more proximal level, smoothing of the bone, skin cover and packing the wound with lint soaked in vinegar. Amputation, he wrote, 'involves a very great risk for patients who often die under the operation . . . but it does not matter whether the remedy is safe enough, since it is the only one'. Celsus, like his Roman colleagues of the time, had use of a wide range of forceps, scalpels and saws and examples of these were found in the ruins of Pompeii, 79 AD (Butler, 1986).

Medical progress was not so rapid over the next 1200 years and the Dark Ages that affected Europe and its medicine are also thought to have affected Indian and Chinese medicine, as there are few accounts of any progress from these areas during this period.

The Middle Ages

During the fourteenth century the numbers of amputees increased due to leprosy and the invention of gunpowder in the 1340s (Rang and Thompson, 1981). The use of firearms and cannon left many people injured and the need for surgical intervention increased, leading to the development of battlefield surgery. In the fifteenth century, the surgeons became more specialized and they left the more difficult physical tasks which were dangerous and dirty to a 'rough, uncouth and uneducated group', the barbers. Some barbers became dexterous with the razor, evolving specialized forms of instruments and by the sixteenth century they had become known as barber surgeons.

Ambrose Paré

Ambrose Paré (1510–1590), the great French army surgeon and father of French surgery, came from a family of barber surgeons. Paré practised in the battlefield and described many procedures of amputation surgery, the most noticeable being the reintroduction of the ligature rather than 'hot irons' to control haemorrhage. Paré also described below knee amputations at a level five finger breadths below the knee (Hamby, 1960), spring-loaded artery forceps to assist holding the vessel closed while ligatures were applied (Bennett-Wilson, 1970), the importance of removing all dead tissue, the appropriate site selection for amputation with prosthetic use in mind and reamputation for prosthetic needs. He described patients following amputation 'walking gaily on a wooden leg'. Paré also described the first elbow disarticulation, amputation above the wrist, in 1536, amputations that healed within 2 months (Hamby, 1960), phantom sensations (Sanders, 1985) and he designed several prostheses for both upper and lower limbs.

Following Paré's work, Lowe, a Scottish army surgeon, in 1596 also described the use of ligatures to control haemorrhages and Fabry, a German surgeon described amputation above the diseased part. In 1558, William Clowes described the first above-knee amputation and in 1679, Lowdham and Yonge described an amputation using a single flap to facilitate skin closure (Sanders, 1985) rather than a circular operation as had almost universally been used by British surgeons up to this time (Butler, 1986). In 1768, Ravaton described the first double flap operation but during the eighteenth and nineteenth centuries, surgeons returned to the single flap technique.

In England, the two arts of surgeon and barber surgeon were separated in the late sixteenth century. They continued to be controlled by the Company of Barbers and Surgeons until 1745 when the Company of Surgeons was formed. In 1800 this became known as the Royal College of Surgeons.

The nineteenth century

Surgery at this time had to be fast to lessen the shock caused by haemorrhage and this became an aim in itself (Vitali et al., 1986). Lisfranc (1790–1847), for example, could amputate through the thigh in 10 seconds and Liston (1794–1847) of University College Hospital, London, was so fast that 'the gleam of his knife was followed so instantaneously by the sound of sawing as to make the two actions appear simultaneous'. Sir William Fergusson, professor of surgery at King's College Hospital, London (1808–1877), wrote in 1846 that 'a surgeon of the present day who takes more than 30 seconds to three minutes, except under peculiar circumstances, for the performance of an amputation whether flap or circular, ought not, in my opinion to be taken as an authority on the subject'.

In 1803, Napoleon's surgeon Larrey (1766–1842) described the operations of hip and shoulder disarticulation and in 1824 the first knee disarticulation. In 1815, Lisfranc described the disarticulation of the foot at the tarsometatarsal joint and in 1842 Syme (1799–1870) of Edinburgh described the operation at the ankle joint.

The use of the tourniquet was earlier described by the Greek surgeons but it was not widely accepted until the eighteenth century, providing surgeons with more time to work. Lisfranc and others advocated waiting a few hours until bleeding stopped before closing the wound to avoid developing haematomas and other surgeons used cold water compresses following surgery until the oozing had stopped. The wounds were subsequently closed with adhesive tape to allow some drainage and avoid the introduction of infection.

In 1846, Fergusson described wound closure with adhesive tape, a light lint dressing and a 'roller applied with moderate tightness'. He also advised that the dressing be changed at 24 hours and then daily for 10–15 days and said that 'the custom of covering the stump with a thick dressing is highly objectionable and is a relic of old, ignorant and barberous surgery'. Through the military surgeons of the time, amputation techniques reached the peak of their advancement and perfection prior to anaesthesia (Rang and Thompson, 1981).

Anaesthetic agents started to be used during the 1840s. Wells and Morton used nitrous oxide and ether and Simpson, in 1847, used chloroform. This made the surgery painless and provided the surgeon with more time (Cartwright, 1977). It did, however, increase the risk of sepsis and death as surgery was now possible in cases that had not been previously attempted. With the advent of anaesthesia, percutaneous sutures for wound closure became common practice.

In North America, the Civil War (1861–1865) left 30 000 amputees in the Union Army alone and with this the thrust of prosthetic design and amputation surgery started in earnest in the USA (Sanders, 1985). In Europe, in 1857, Gritti modified the knee operation that had initially been described by Smith in 1843, in which the patella was used as a weight-bearing surface. This operation was again modified by Stoke (1839–1900) in 1870. Cheyne and Burghard in 1900, however, wrote that 'it does not present any advantage which counterbalances the increased time and patience required for its proper performance' and even today it remains a controversial operation.

During the Crimean War (1854–1856), Florence Nightingale, a nurse from St Thomas' Hospital in London, succeeded in bringing 'scientific cleanliness to the military situation, reducing infection and replacing the hospital chaos with orderliness' (Rang and Thompson, 1981). Post-operative wound infection leading to sepsis was frequent at this time and devastating. A remark from this period said 'it was much less dangerous to have a thigh amputation by gunfire on the battle field, than by a surgeon' (Schmuker, 1774).

Cleanliness, so important to early Greek surgeons, was far from the surgical practice of the nineteenth century. There were many reports of 'dirty white aprons' and public surgery. Surgeons operated without gowns and gloves and there were reports from the 1870–1880s in the USA, of sutures being carried in button holes and even in the surgeon's mouth (Vitali *et al.*, 1986). In 1867, Lord Lister, a surgeon who held the chair of clinical surgery at King's College Hospital, London, started to use carbolic-impregnated lint as an antiseptic in surgery and to use antiseptic techniques. His techniques reduced operative mortality by 66% and virtually eliminated general sepsis which had so often caused death earlier (Cartwright, 1977). Lister's principles were adopted by the US Army in 1877 and by the American Surgical Association in 1883.

The Germans in the Franco Prussian war of 1870 continued this thrust forward, recognizing that dirty hands on dressings was the most potent source of infection. Sterilization by heat and the use of operating gowns and caps and face masks (Cartwright, 1977) changed surgeons from using antiseptic to aseptic techniques. Aseptic techniques now superseded antiseptics. Rubber gloves were not introduced until the beginning of the twentieth century.

In 1895 the hemipelvectomy operation was first described by Girard of Switzerland and in 1909 Ransohoff described the operation in the USA. Advancements in the late nineteenth century were due to anaesthetics, antiseptics and aseptic techniques.

Recent history

Before the First World War (1914–1918) in Europe, amputation surgery and surgery generally was improving. In 1928, Alexander Fleming of St Mary's Hospital, London, discovered penicillin and by the 1940s it was being manufactured in large quantities in both the UK and USA. Also in 1938, bacterostatic drugs such as the sulphonamides were discovered. The problems of sepsis that earlier amputation surgeons had encountered were now conquered.

Prosthetics were, however, not so advanced at this time and the limb makers required conical stumps in which the muscle was allowed to retract, to fit the plug-type socket of the day. The bulbous stumps of Syme and through knee amputations were taboo and so simple flaps and guillotine type amputations were the most common (Vitali *et al.*, 1986). However, surgeons found that the stumps often became ulcerated, oedematous or cold and painful. In 1952, following the work of Dr Felix Mondry, practice changed and these symptoms were corrected by the myoplastic type of operation, where opposite muscle groups are stitched over the end of the stump at the correct tension in order to produce a stump that is physiologically stable and in which the vascular dynamics are efficient. The history of amputation surgery closely follows the history of surgery itself. Once asepsis and anaesthetics were introduced and the morbidity and mortality of operation reduced, the techniques of amputation surgery were able to develop further. Some techniques, however, have followed those laid down in ancient Greek times. Today's amputation techniques are discussed in Chapter 5.

PROSTHETIC HISTORY

The word **prosthetic** is derived from the Greek word meaning addition.

Early history

Very early records of prosthetic replacement have been found. For example, descriptions dating from 3500 to 1800 BC have been found in India (Sanders, 1985), and in Europe in the fifth century BC, Herodotus described a wooden foot being fitted following an amputation. There are also other examples: a prosthetic leg dating from 300 BC and made from wood with bronze and iron was found in a tomb in Capua, Italy (Vitali et al., 1986); a prosthetic hand belonging to a Roman General dating from 218 BC and an iron hand from the Second Punic War (218–202 BC) (McCord, 1963).

The Middle Ages

In the Middle Ages, prostheses were chiefly made for the below-knee amputee. They were made from wood for the peasants or poor and from metal for the wealthy, and little consideration was paid to function or cosmesis. The iron 'additions' for the wealthy were made by the armourers to look like armour and were used to hide the amputees' disability, a point of weakness in combat. They were extremely heavy but this was not a problem as the knights were either carried or rode horses. Those who were unable to obtain wooden legs resorted to hopping with crutches or propelling themselves on moveable benches. Gradually prostheses became more sophisticated. For example, the Stibbert collection in Florence includes many examples of fifteenth and sixteenth-century prostheses, including the Alt-Ruppin hand (1400 AD) which consists of a moveable wrist, a rigid thumb fixed in opposition and flexible fingers operating in pairs. They were flexed manually and locked into position in a ratchet mechanism (Vitali *et al.*, 1986).

Developments continued, and in 1696 the Dutch surgeon Verduin described a below-knee prosthesis with a copper socket lined with a leather thigh corset and a locked knee, external articulating hinges and a wooden foot. Ankle and foot joints were developed during the eighteenth century by Grossmith (1750) and Ravadon (1775) and, in 1786, Bruninghausen developed an above-knee and below-knee prosthesis with a rigid ankle, similar in principle to the modern solid ankle cushion heel (SACH) design of foot. Gavin Ilson of Edinburgh, at the end of the eighteenth century, fabricated a prosthesis of hardened leather with a knee joint which could flex in sitting but was designed with a stiff knee joint and an ischial seat for walking.

The nineteenth century

In 1800, James Potts described a wooden leg with a synchronous motion of the prosthetic knee and ankle, a steel knee and a wooden ankle joint. Cords from the knee controlled the ankle movement allowing the toe to clear the ground in the swing phase. Historically the leg became known as the 'Anglesey' leg as it was worn by the Marquis of Anglesey in 1816 after he lost a leg at the Battle of Waterloo (1815). It was also nicknamed the 'clapper leg' because during locomotion it made a clapping noise. The design, with some modifications, was used by the British until the First World War. In 1839, the Potts or Anglesey leg was taken to the USA by Selpho (an apprentice of Potts) and modified by the addition of a rubber sole and a rubber plate to the ankle. Palmer again modified the design and patented it in 1846 when it became known as the 'American' leg.

In 1810, Von Heine of Würzburg designed an artificial leg which had a ball joint at the ankle and was suspended from the trunk by a corset (Sanders, 1985). A year later, Professor Antenrieth used waist belts and shoulder straps over the opposite shoulder to suspend wooden legs and in 1831 Goyrand described the concept of using the ischial tuberosity for weight bearing. The first year that rubber was used in the field of prosthetics was 1839 and in 1842, Martin and Charrière introduced an automatic passive control of the knee in extension by placing the knee centre posterior to the central axis of the prosthesis.

In 1818, Baliff, a Berlin dentist, introduced the use of the trunk and shoulder girdle muscles as a source of power to flex or extend the fingers following an arm amputation. In 1844, Van Peetersen (McCord, 1963), a Dutch sculptor, used Baliff's principle for a prosthesis that flexed at the elbow for the upper arm amputee.

The Crimean War in Europe led to a number of prosthetic advances. The Comte de Beaufort of France designed two simple wooden legs and demonstrated an arm in which elbow flexion was activated by the pressure of a lever against the chest. In 1867, he also published a design of an operating harness and an automatic knee lock similar to that used today. In 1858, Dr Bly of New York introduced a ball and socket design for the ankle joint and in 1859, Marks described a leg with knee, ankle and toe movements and the first rubber foot (McCord, 1963).

During the American Civil War in 1861, J.E. Hangar, one of the first Southerns to lose a leg (Bennett-Wilson, 1970), opened a prosthetic company in Virginia, USA, and developed rubber bumpers to control plantar and dorsiflexion (McCord, 1963). In 1863, an American, Parmalee, patented a suction socket but it failed to find acceptance until the Germans reintroduced the concept in Europe following the Second World War. Aluminium instead of steel was used in a prosthesis by Hermann of Prague in 1865 and a year later Clasen described the first functional heavy duty hand that was capable of holding heavy objects. In 1880 the 'laminated' foot was patented.

From 1870 in the USA, limbs were issued free to war veterans and replaced every 5 years. This was changed in 1891 to a new limb being issued every 3 years and free transportation to and from the manufacturers was also included.

Recent history

In 1912 three new prosthetic designs emerged. Firstly, in the UK Desoutter produced the first all-aluminium prosthesis with the pelvic suspension concept and secondly, Carnes produced the Sunday or parlor arm which was a versatile upper limb prosthesis allowing the fingers to flex, the wrist to pronate and supinate, extend and flex and the elbow to flex and extend. Supination was synchronized with flexion and pronation with extension but the device lacked durability (Rang and Thompson, 1981). Thirdly, D.W. Dorrance developed the first split hook for the upper limb, of which a refined design is still used today. Beaufort designed a foot with a rocking sole which, following modification, became known as the Dollinger foot and was widely used in the First World War.

The First World War left more amputees than previously known from warfare. Surgical advances were such that many more soldiers survived the horrors of war. In Europe there were 100 000 amputees, in the UK 42 000 and in the USA a smaller number of 4403 amputees (Sanders, 1985). In Britain, war amputees received pensions that were graded according to their limb loss. For example, an amputee who had lost his leg at the hip joint received the largest pension and the prosthesis was coded number 1. A below-knee amputee lost less, received a smaller pension and the prosthesis was coded number 8 on the scale. These codes are still used in British prosthetic prescription and are given in Chapter 12. Developments in the UK prosthetic service at this time are discussed in Chapter 11.

An engineer and surgeon team from Belfast, Pringle and Kirk (James and Orr, 1986) developed an arm in 1918 which had a four-finger grip and in 1921 developed a 'safety knee', a design which was moving towards that of a 'four bar linkage' joint of today. There were few advances in prosthetics between the two wars due to a lack of incentive and the Depression. However, a prosthetist and surgeon team from Denver, USA, Thomas and Hadden, emphasized that 'fit and alignment of a prosthesis were the most critical factors in the success of any limb and better results were found if the prosthetist and surgeon worked together' (Bennett-Wilson, 1970).

The Second World War (1939–1945) produced a large number of young amputees, providing the incentive for another developmental thrust. The numbers were, however, not as large as in the First World War due to the availability of sulphonamides and penicillin and improved surgical care. In the USA a prosthetic research programme was initiated in 1945 and in 1947 the Veterans Administration was established with a prosthetic research laboratory in New York. Also, at the University of California, research studies were started at Berkeley of the lower limb and at Los Angeles of the upper limb (Sanders, 1985). In Canada during the post-war period, the Department of Veterans' Affairs was established at Sunnybrook Hospital, Toronto, and following the thalidomide disaster of 1963 this was extended to include Montreal, Winnipeg and Fredericton (Rang and Thompson, 1981). These programmes in both the USA and Canada were co-ordinated by the Committee on Prosthetic Research and Development.

In the UK, with the inception of the National Health Service in 1948, the 30 000 civilian amputees joined with the 45 000 war pensioner amputees in becoming entitled to free artificial limbs.

Prosthetic developments continued. For example, in 1954, Colin McLaurin of Sunnybrook Hospital, Toronto, developed the Canadian hip disarticulation prosthesis and in 1956 the solid ankle cushion heel foot (SACH) was developed at the Biomechanics Laboratory of the University of California. In 1958, Berlemont of France introduced the concept of immediate post-surgical fitting of a prosthesis and a major breakthrough for the below-knee amputee, the patella tendon bearing (PTB) below-knee prosthesis, was introduced by Radcliffe and Foort at the University of California at Berkeley in 1959.

In 1960, Stewart of the Vickers Company developed the Hydra Cadence leg which achieved knee stability by weight bearing through the ball of the foot. Plantaflexion was controlled by a hydraulic cylinder and the knee and ankle movements were co-ordinated during the swing phase to give greater clearance (Sanders, 1985). In 1963, Fajal of France introduced a PTB prosthesis with supracondylar suspension, the prosthese tibiale supracondylienne (PTS). In 1966, Dr Gotz-Gerd Kuhn of Munster Germany developed the wedge suspension socket for the below-knee amputee, the Kondyler bettung Munster (KBM), and the PTS was introduced by Marshall and Nitschke to the USA. A suction PTB prosthesis was developed in Sweden in 1969 and a pneumatic piston cylinder was developed at the University of California in 1970. Another major breakthrough for modern prosthetics occurred in 1971 when endoskeletal prostheses were introduced by the Otto Bock company which consisted of an adjustable tubular structure, which was encased in a foam and elastic stocking hose.

The thalidomide tragedy of 1959–1960 provided another thrust of incentive for governments to put money into prosthetic research (Bennett-Wilson, 1970). In 1959, the American Orthopaedic Appliance and Limb Manufacturers' Association changed its name to become the American Orthotics and Prosthetics Association (AOPA). In 1965 in the USA the Medicine Bill was passed allowing people over 65 years of age artificial limbs at a minimal cost. In 1970, an international prosthetic and orthotic society was formed to improve communication between research and clinical practice worldwide. This is the International Society of Prosthetics and Orthotics (ISPO).

The field of prosthetics is currently changing rapidly as new materials become available and are applied to the field. Changes are also occurring as techniques of casting change and the prosthetists' training and attitudes also change. The prostheses that are commonly prescribed today are discussed in Chapter 12.

REFERENCES

Bennett-Wilson, A. (1970) Limb prosthetics – 1970. *Artificial Limbs*, **14**, 1–52.
Butler, C.M. (1986) The vascular amputee, MS Thesis, University of London.

Cartwright, F.F. (1977) The birth of scientific medicine, in *A Social History of Medicine*, Longman Group Ltd, London, pp. 131–150.

Hamby, W.B. (1960) *The Case Reports and Autopsy Records of Ambroise Paré*, Charles C. Thomas, London.

Isherwood, P.A. (1980) The controlled pressure distribution system for prosthetic casting, (PhD Thesis), University of London.

James, W.V. and Orr, J.F. (1986) The Pringle and Kirk four bar crossed linkage and the 'safety knee'. *Prosthet. Orthot. Int.*, **10**, 23–26.

McCord, C.P. (1963) Cork legs and iron hands: the early history of artificial limbs. *Indust. Med. Surg.* **32**, 102–112.

Rang, M. and Thompson, G.H. (1981) History of amputation and prostheses, in *Amputation Surgery and Rehabilitation – the Toronto Experience* (ed. J.P. Kostuik), Churchill Livingstone, New York, pp. 1–12.

Ruffer, M.A. (1921) In *The Palacopathology of Ancient Egypt*. Chicago University Press, Chicago.

Sanders, G.T. (1985) History, in *Lower Limb Amputations: A Guide to Rehabilitation*, F.A. Davis Co., Philadelphia, pp. 13–33.

Schmuker, J.C. (1774) *Chirurgische Wahrnehmugen*, Berlin.

Vitali, M., Robinson, K.P., Andrews, B.G., Harris, E.E. and Redhead, R.G. (1986) A brief historical survey, in *Amputations and Prostheses*, Baillière Tindall, London, pp. 1–10.

2

Amputation data – the background to practice

INTRODUCTION

Today the economic climate is such that unit policies, practices, financial statements and equipment provision are made on the basis of data collection. Data regarding amputation numbers, levels, supply and use, for example, are therefore becoming increasingly important for comparison and audit purposes and this chapter summarizes some current data on this subject.

AMPUTATION TRENDS

At the beginning of this century, the majority of amputations resulted from the traumas of war. For example, during the First World War, 25 000 amputees were treated at one prosthetic centre in the UK, Roehampton. Following the Second World War this figure increased, though not so dramatically and by 1945 there were 45 000 war pensioners in the UK. As war pensioners died, the numbers being cared for in the UK gradually fell (English and Dean, 1980). Since the Second World War, the resulting cause of amputation has changed. Today the majority of amputations are due to vascular insufficiency and not trauma. This change in referral from trauma to vascular disease has seen an increase of referrals to our prosthetic centres over the last 30 years as surgical practice, technology and life expectancy have increased. In 1961, the number of patients referred to centres for prosthetic prescription in the UK was 3500. In 1970 the figure had risen to 4559 and by 1985 to 5461 (Ham *et al.*, 1989a). Many amputees in the UK, as in other western countries, are either physically, medically or mentally unsuitable for a limb and are therefore not referred. It has been estimated that the true amputation figure is twice the number that receives prostheses from the centres, that is approximately 8–11 000 per annum (Dormandy and Thomas, 1988).

The population of the UK has increased by three million since 1961 but the amputations for vascular disease have doubled. From the USA, similar increases are reported. In 1965 there were 33 000 primary amputees and by 1971 this figure had increased to 43 000. The total number of amputees (primary and established) recorded through prosthetic shops in the USA was 311 000 in 1971 and had increased to 500 000 in 1980 (Banerjee, 1982). In 1981 the UK amputation rate figure of 34 per 100 000 population was identical to that of North America (Butler, 1986).

In other western countries similar trends have been observed. In Sweden, the population almost doubled between 1910 and 1979 and yet the amputation rate increased more than 10 times (Liedberg and Persson, 1982). The amputation rate in 1947 in Gothenburg, Sweden, was six per 100 000 population. This had increased to 17 per 100 000 in 1962 and 41 per 100 000 population in 1977 (Renström, 1981). Similar trends have also been reported from Denmark and Finland. In Finland in 1972 the amputation rate in the Helsinki area was 15.4 per 100 000 population. By 1984 this figure had increased to 32.5 per 100 000 population (Pohjolainen and Alaranta, 1988).

DISEASE

Today the major causes of amputation are vascular disease, diabetes, trauma, tumour and congenital deformity. The major causes vary in different parts of the world. For example, in the west, it is vascular disease and diabetes but in the Third World it is trauma. In England and Wales, the percentage of amputations for vascular disease has increased to 54%, diabetes remains static and the percentage of amputations for trauma has decreased (Ham et al., 1989a). In Scotland the percentage of amputations for vascular disease is higher, 65% (Knight and Urquhart, 1989).

Similar data are seen in Sweden. Between 1926 and 1930, 67% of all amputations were due to trauma and 2% due to vascular disease. By 1955 the cause had completely reversed; trauma accounted for 29% and vascular disease for 57% (Hansson, 1964). In Finland similar pattern changes are seen. In 1975, the figure for vascular disease was 75% and trauma 12%. By 1984 the figures for vascular disease had increased to 88% and for trauma had fallen to 2% (Pohjolainen and Alaranta, 1988).

In Denmark, vascular disease accounts for 61% of all amputations (Ebskov, 1988).

In the USA between 1961 and 1963, the percentage of amputations for vascular disease was 58% and this rose to 70% in 1973–1974. The trauma figure was 33% in 1961–1963 and fell to 22% in 1973–1974. Diabetes accounts for between 33 and 69% of amputations in a number of reported series (Sanders, 1986). However, problems of accurate statistical collection apply in the USA as they do in the UK because the figures have been collected at prosthetic shops and centres and not at the operating or inpatient source. Many large studies from the USA do not address themselves specifically to the diabetic question. However, diabetics have their first amputation at an earlier age than non-diabetics (Butler, 1986).

Narang reported an increase in the percentage of amputations for trauma in India since 1954. Trauma accounted for 67% of all amputations between 1954 and 1978 (Narang and Jape, 1982) and for 82% in a more recent study (Narang et al., 1984). From another Third World country, Burma, the picture is different. Forty-seven per cent of all lower limb amputations were due to trauma and 41% due to disease (Pe, 1988). In Hong Kong, 26% of all lower limb amputations reported were due to trauma, 31% to vascular disease and diabetes, but the largest percentage (35%) was due to infection (Chan et al., 1984). In Japan, the main cause of amputation is trauma. Vascular disease accounts for approximately 20% of all amputations but this figure is rising (Dazai, 1988).

AGE

In the west the general age of the population and that of the amputee is rising. In the UK in 1984, more than 75% of all amputees referred to the prosthetic centres were over 60 years of age (McColl, 1986) whereas in 1961 this figure was only 50%. From Sweden a 4 year increase was reported in mean age at amputation between 1955 and 1962 (Hansson, 1964) and an 8 year increase in the mean age between 1949 and 1979 (Renström, 1981). In a Finnish study the majority of amputees were over 60 years of age. The mean male age at amputation was 71 years and the mean female age was 79.6 years (Pohjolainen and Alaranta, 1988).

In the Third World, the average age of the amputee is much lower. In Burma, a mean age of 31 years was reported (Pe, 1988), in Hong Kong, 39 years (Chan et al., 1984) and in India, 25 years (Narang and Jape, 1982). The largest group of amputees in Japan is between the ages of

18–24 years (Dazai, 1988). An Australian study reported that the mean age of the lower limb amputee in that country was 53 years between 1981 and 1985 (Jones, 1989).

MALE : FEMALE RATIO

The reported male:female ratios from the UK, USA and Scandinavia are 2:1 and this has not altered over the last 20 years. In Scotland, the same ratio was found to be 3:2 in those under 75 years, equal in the 74–84 year age group and $1:3\frac{1}{2}$ in those over 84 years (Knight and Urquhart, 1989). In Burma the male:female ratio is reported as 4:1 (Pe, 1988) and in Japan 5:1 (Dazai, 1988).

UPPER:LOWER LIMB RATIO

Reports from both the UK and USA are of a ratio of upper to lower limb amputees that is widening. In 1961 in the UK the ratio was 1:11 and in the USA in the same year 1:6. In 1973 in the USA this had increased to 1:11 (Sanders, 1986) and in 1982 in the UK it was reported to be 1:26. In the underdeveloped world the ratios were opposite. In India and Hong Kong, the upper to lower limb ratio is 2:1 (Narang and Jape, 1982; Chan, 1984) and in Burma the figure is 4:1 (Pe, 1988). In Japan it is 1:2 (Dazai, 1988).

LEVELS OF AMPUTATION

It is now well established that saving the knee joint increases the amputee's rehabilitation potential. A below-knee (BK) to above-knee (AK) amputation ratio of $1:2\frac{1}{2}$ is said to be the minimum acceptable for units providing a lower limb service. In reviewing data over the last 30 years, it was seen that this ratio is rarely reached (Dormandy and Thomas, 1988). Between 1981 and 1985 in England, Wales and Northern Ireland, the AK amputations remained at a mean of 49% and the BK amputations at a mean of 41% (Ham et al., 1989a). In Scotland, the reported figure for BK amputations was 53%, and 40% for AK amputations. In 1976, a 75% BK figure was reported from an informed centre (Robinson, 1976). In the USA generally, the AK figure fell between 1961–1963 and 1973–1974 from 44 to 33% and the BK figure

15

increased from 37 to 54% (Sanders, 1986). From Canada in 1975, an AK level of 45% and BK level of 38% was reported (Banerjee, 1982). The ratio of AK to BK amputations can be reversed when a positive approach is taken (Little *et al.*, 1973). For example, between 1956 and 1962 the AK:BK ratio reported was 146:19 and following changes in 1962 it was reported as 4:1. A UK centre reports the reduction of AK amputations from 88 to 33%, by gaining surgical interest and implementing a team approach (Ham *et al.*, 1987). Similar results have also been reported from the USA. In 1960–1963 the figure of AK amputations was 69.3%. With the change in practice between 1964 and 1968, this AK figure had fallen to 17%, more knees having been saved (Sarmiento *et al.*, 1970).

From India, Narang *et al.* (1984) reported a BK figure of 61.5% and 25% at the AK level. In Hong Kong, BK amputations accounted for 60% and AK amputations for 25% of the lower limb amputation total (Chan *et al.*, 1984). This is similar in Burma, where BK amputations account for 65% and AK amputations for 28% of the lower limb total (Pe, 1988).

It has been reported that smokers are more likely to have an amputation at the AK level than non-smokers (Stewart, 1987) and the population of smokers at the time of amputation is higher in patients with peripheral vascular disease than in the general population (Knight and Urquhart, 1989).

HEALING

Healing by first intention or primary healing is generally regarded as occurring within 30 days of surgery. Delayed healing or by secondary intention describes healing which takes longer than this but without surgical intervention. From the Dundee Limb Fitting Centre, the best results are recorded, 66% by primary healing and 28% by delayed healing, a total of 94% (Cummings *et al.*, 1987). The remaining 6% underwent a wedge resection (local refashioning) before healing at the below-knee level occurred. Renström (1981) described primary healing in below-knee amputation in 69.4% of patients at 6 weeks post-surgery, which including those with delayed healing (18.8%), brought the total to 88%. Another report described primary healing in 70% of patients with delayed healing in 15% – making a total of 85% (Dormandy and Thomas, 1988).

AMPUTATION OF THE CONTRALATERAL LEG – THE BILATERAL AMPUTEE

As the majority of amputations in the west are carried out for vascular disease, a generalized degenerative condition, it is not surprising that patients also lose their remaining leg. The period between the loss of the first and second limb varies considerably in the published material and this is due to both the nature of the disease and the varieties of surgical practices. Data from the National Danish Amputation Register (Ebskov, 1988) show that 19% of amputees lose their second leg within 6 months of the first amputation; data from London show 37% (Butler, 1986). The figure is a little more encouraging from the USA where it is reported that 10% lose their second leg in 1 year, 20% in 2 years and 33% within 5 years (Sanders, 1986). From an Australian study, it was reported that 24% of amputees lost their second leg or died within 5 years (Little et al., 1973). In a recent Scottish survey, 2% lost their second leg 6 months after their first amputation, 5% in 1 year and 7% in 18 months (Knight and Urquhart, 1989). The severity of the disease and the timing of the first amputation vary enormously and currently no baseline for data collection is available. However, the importance of saving the knee joint whenever possible is emphasized.

MORTALITY

Many authors describe high mortality figures for these vascular patients and this is considerably higher than the equivalent general population matched for age and sex distribution (Butler, 1986). For example, 53% survival at 20 months (Renström, 1981), 50% survival at 3 years (Britton and Barrie, 1987), 41% survival at 2 years (Kihn et al., 1972), 53% survival at 3 years (Little et al., 1974) and 58% survival rate at 2 years post-amputation (Hansson, 1964) have been reported. In a Scottish survey a mortality rate of 17% at 1 year and 28% at 2 years post-amputation was reported (Knight and Urquhart, 1989). As primary amputations are carried out at different times in each patient's disease pattern, it is not surprising that these figures vary. Life expectancy for the vascular amputee is undoubtedly poor and it is imperative that rehabilitation and successful return to the community is achieved as soon as possible so that the remaining months are not wasted in hospital.

HOSPITALIZATION PERIOD

In general the hospital stay reported for the below-knee amputee is longer than that for the above-knee amputee. Renström (1981) described a mean in-patient stay for surgery and full rehabilitation of 59 days for a prosthesis for a below-knee group. Fifty-nine days is echoed by Britton and Barrie (1987) following successful below-knee amputation. Haynes and Middleton (1981) described a mean of 65 days and Harris *et al.* (1974) a mean of 57.6 days. Ebskov (1983) reported a 40% discharge rate at the end of the first post-operative month and 75% at the end of 2 months. Robinson (1976), in a specialized unit, quotes a mean of 3 months and Weaver and Marshall (1973) quote 83 days for below-knee amputees and 56 days for above-knee amputees. Kald *et al.* (1989), from Sweden, reported a hospital stay as long as 184 days from a district hospital, a non-specialist centre.

Malone *et al.* (1981) describe the mean day stay before and after a change in the rehabilitation programme, making it more intense and economic. Before changes, the mean day stay was 68 days and following the changes it fell to 38 days. In a UK study before an active team approach was implemented, patients were discharged at a mean of 71 days without being fully rehabilitated on a prosthesis. With the implementation of the team approach and discharge when rehabilitation was complete, hospital stay fell to 51 days (Ham *et al.*, 1987). Unfortunately with changes in staff, the day stay has increased to 73 days (Ham *et al.*, 1989b).

PROSTHETIC USE

The majority of amputations in the west today are for vascular disease, and therefore the use of follow-up studies in the use of a prosthesis will show a decrease in the majority of cases, the longer the review period from the patient's first amputation, as the patient's condition deteriorates. Britton and Barrie (1987) describe 84% of below-knee amputees and 72% of above-knee amputees using their prosthesis at follow-up. Dormandy and Thomas (1988) described prosthetic use for the below-knee amputee with full mobility that ranged from 30 to 85% and partial mobility that ranged from 9 to 42%. For the above-knee amputee these figures were 11–36% and 9–74%, respectively. Steinberg *et al.* (1985) described a study of follow-up at 22 months after surgery. Seventy-three per cent of below-knee amputees were using their prosthesis full time and 25% part of the time. Fifty per cent of above-knee amputees were using them full time and of the bilaterals, 33% were using them full time. Steinberg felt that age was not a major factor in prosthetic use but that concurrent medical disease or mental deterioration was. A Scottish survey reported that 93% of all patients seen at limb fitting centres were supplied with prostheses and 62% of the patients used their prosthesis all day every day, 15% used them for half a day and 4% for half of the week. Once the general pattern of use was established, it was found to be sustained over the review period of 18 months (Knight and Urquhart, 1989). Christensen (1976) reported that it took 17.7 weeks for a below-knee amputee to walk independently with a prosthesis and 19.5 weeks for an above-knee amputee to walk from the time of surgery. He also reported that a quarter of those fitted with a prosthesis did not wear them. In a UK study, functional prosthetic use at one year was poor (33%) when patients did not receive their prosthesis while an in-patient. Once they were fully rehabilitated in hospital before discharge, the functional use at one year increased to a mean of 88% (range 78–94%) (Ham et al., 1989b).

SOCIAL DEPRIVATION

In a London survey it was found that elements of social deprivation, for example poor housing, lack of adequate heating, poverty and unemployment, are important factors in the natural history of ischaemic disease leading to limb amputation (Butler, 1986).

RESULTS OF A LONDON SURVEY 1981–1983

During the period 1981–1983, Butler reviewed patients from London who were referred to the Roehampton and Stanmore prosthetic centres. The numbers accounted for 10% of the total vascular amputee referrals in the UK and 41% had had previous vascular surgery on the side of the amputation. In 36% of patients this was within less than 3 months of the amputation. Of the amputees aged between 50 and 60 years, 61% had had previous vascular surgery and 12% had previously had two or more procedures. Non-diabetic patients had more above-knee amputations (44%) than below-knee amputations (42%), whereas diabetic cases accounted for 26% at the above-knee level and 54% at the below-knee level. Sixteen per cent of all the patients required more than one amputation to achieve healing.

Many of the published studies come from centres where there is an interest in the subject. However, from Butler's data the work of different hospitals was compared. Fifty-eight hospitals referred patients following amputation for limb fitting, and 18 hospitals referred more than 20 amputees. The hospitals were divided into three groups; London teaching hospitals, university hospitals with teaching hospital links and district general hospitals (DGH). The teaching hospital patients were younger and there was a larger percentage of diabetics. The teaching and university hospital patients had undergone a higher percentage of vascular surgery procedures prior to amputation than the DGHs. The percentage of below-knee amputees varied from between 37 and 85% at teaching hospitals, 20 and 50% at university hospitals and 11 and 75% at DGHs. The failure rate of amputations at these hospitals was between 10 and 17% and did not relate to the numbers of below-knee amputations being performed (Butler, 1986).

SUMMARY

1. The number of elderly people in the west is increasing and the number of amputees is increasing because of this.
2. In the west there is an increase in the number of patients requiring amputation for vascular disease and a decrease in those requiring amputation for trauma.
3. The age of the western world's population is increasing and medically there is now a more active attitude to the aged. The economic status of the amputee has improved. The governments are now providing prostheses free, therefore more are being fitted than in earlier years.
4. The male:female ratio of 2:1 remains static.
5. The ratio between lower and upper limb amputations is increasing.
6. The UK national AK:BK ratio is approximately equal. In the USA there are reports of more below-knee amputations. In an interested centre, it is very possible to increase the numbers of below-knee amputations.
7. Many amputees lose their second leg within 12 months of losing their first, so preservation of the knee joint is vital to maximize their rehabilitation potential.
8. The hospital stay from amputation to full rehabilitation is approximately 51 days. Improving the practice will reduce the mean day stay. Local goal setting should be encouraged.
9. Primary healing for below-knee amputees, especially in trained hands, is highly possible.

10. Prosthetic use at follow-up is good where supply and rehabilitation are good.

REFERENCES

Banerjee, S.N. (1982) Limb amputation – incidence, cause and prevention, in *Rehabilitation Management of Amputees* (Ed. S.N. Banerjee), pp. 1–10. Rehabilitation Medicine Library, Baltimore.

Britton, P.J. and Barrie, W.W. (1987) Amputation in the diabetic: 10-year experience in a district general hospital. *Ann. R. Coll. Surg. (Eng.)*, **69**, 127–129.

Butler, C.M. (1986) The vascular amputee, MS Thesis, University of London.

Chan, K.M., Cheung, D., Sher, A., Leung, P.C., Fuk, T. and Lee, J. (1984) A 24 year survey of amputees in Hong Kong. *Prosthet. Orthot. Int.*, **8**, 155–158.

Christensen, S. (1976) Lower extremity amputations in the county of Aalborg 1961–1971. *Acta Orthop. Scand.*, **47**, 329–334.

Cummings, J.G.R., Jain, A.S., Walker, W.F., Spence, V.A. and Stewart, C. (1987) Fate of the vascular patient after lower limb amputation. *Lancet*, **ii**, 613–615.

Dazai, H. (1988) Medical rehabilitation, in *Rehabilitation in Japan*, pp. 77–105. Japanese Society for Rehabilitation of the Disabled.

Dormandy, J.A. and Thomas, P.R.S. (1988) What is the natural of a critically ischaemic patient with and without a leg? in *Limb Salvage and Amputation for Vascular Disease* (Ed. R.M. Greenhalgh, C.W. Jamieson, and A.N. Nicolaides), Saunders, London, pp. 11–26.

Ebskov, B. (1983) Choice of level in lower extremity amputation – nationwide survey. *Prosthet. Orthot. Int.*, **7**, 58–60.

Ebskov, B. (1988) Trends in lower extremity amputation (Denmark 1978–1983), in *Amputation Surgery and Lower Limb Prosthetics* (Ed. G. Murdoch), Blackwell Scientific, Oxford, pp. 3–8.

English, A.W.G. and Dean, G.A.A. (1980) The artificial limb service. *Health Trends*, **12**, 77–82.

Ham, R.O., Regan, J.M. and Roberts, V.C. (1987) Evaluation of introducing the team approach to the care of the amputee: the Dulwich Study. *Prosthet. Orthot. Int.*, **11**, 25–30.

Ham, R.O., Luff, R. and Roberts, V.C. (1989a) A five-year review of referrals for prosthetic treatment in England, Wales and Northern Ireland 1981–1985. *Health Trends*, **21**, 3–6.

Ham, R., Sweet, A. and Roberts, V.C. (1989b) The Dulwich Study: A Team Approach update (in press).

Hansson, J. (1964) The leg amputee: a clinical follow up study. *Acta Orth. Scand.*, Suppl. 69.

Harris, P.L., Read, F., Eardley, A., Charlesworth, D., Wakefield, J. and Sellwood, R.A. (1974) The fate of elderly amputees. *Br. J. Surg.*, **61**, 665–668.

Haynes, I.G. and Middleton, M.D. (1981) Amputation for peripheral vascular disease: experience of a district general hospital. *Ann. R. Coll. Surg. (Eng.)*, **63**, 342–344.

Jones, L.E. (1989) Prosthetic limb use in Australia 1981–1985 under the free limb scheme. *Prosthet. Orthot. Int.*, **13**, 76–81.

Kald, A., Carlsson, R. and Nilsson, E. (1989) Major amputation in a defined population: incidence, mortality, and results of treatment. *Br. J. Surg.*, **76**, 308–310.

Kihn, R.B., Warren, R. and Beebe, G.W. (1972) The geriatric amputee. *Ann. Surg.*, **176**, 305–314.

Knight, P. and Urquhart, J. (1989) in *Outcomes of Artificial Lower Limb Fitting in Scotland*. I.S.D. Publications, Scottish Health Service.

Liedberg, E. and Persson, B.M. (1982) Increased incidence of lower limb amputation for arterial occlusive disease, in *Amputation för Kärlsjukdom, Lunds Universitet*, pp. 1.2–1.12.

Little, J.M., Petritsi-Jones, D., Zylstra, P., Williams, R. and Kerr, C. (1973) A survey of amputations for degenerative vascular disease. *Med. J. Aust.*, 17 Feb., 329–334.

Little, J.M., Petritsi-Jones, D. and Kerr, C. (1974) Vascular amputees: a study in disappointment. *Lancet*, **i**, 793–795.

Malone, J.M., Moore, W., Leal, J.M. and Childers, S.J. (1981) Rehabilitation for lower extremity amputation. *Arch. Surg.*, **116**, 93–98.

McColl, I. (1986) *Review of Artificial Limb and Appliance Centre Services*. London, DHSS.

Narang, I.C. and Jape, V.C. (1982) Retrospective study of 14 400 civilian disabled (new) treated over 25 years at an Artificial Limb centre. *Prosthet. Orthot. Int.*, **6**, 10–16.

Narang, I.C., Mathur, B.P., Singh, P. and Jape, V.C. (1984) Functional capabilities of Lower Limb amputees. *Prosthet. Orthot. Int.*, **8**, 43–51.

Pe, H. (1988) A 15 year survey of Burmese amputees. *Prosthet. Orthot. Int.*, **2**, 65–72.

Pohjolainen, T. and Alaranta, H. (1988) Lower limb amputation in Southern Finland 1984–1985. *Prosthet. Orthot. Int.*, **12**, 9–18.

Pohjolainen, T., Alaranta, H. and Wilström, J. (1989) Primary survival and prosthetic fitting of lower limb amputees. *Prosthet. Orthot. Int.*, **13**, 63–69.

Renström, P. (1981) A follow up study of 200 below knee amputations amputated between 1973–1977, in *The Below Knee Amputee*, pp. 7–25. MD Thesis, Gothenburg, Sweden.

Robinson, K.P. (1976) Long posterior flap amputation in geriatric patients with ischaemic disease. *Ann. R. Coll. Surg. (Eng.)*, **58**, 440–451.

Sanders, G.T. (1986) Statistics, in *Lower Limb Amputations: a Guide to Rehabilitation*, pp. 35–55. FA Davis Co. Philadelphia.

Sarmiento, A., May, B.J., Sinclair, W.F., McCollough, N.C. and Williams, E.M. (1970) Lower extremity amputation. *Clin. Orthop. Relat. Res.*, **68**, 22–31.

Steinberg, F.U., Sunwoo, L. and Roettger, R.F. (1985) Prosthetic rehabilitation of geriatric amputee patients: a follow up study. *Arch. Phys. Med. Rehabil.*, **66**, 742–745.

Stewart, C.P.U. (1987) The influence of smoking on the level of lower limb amputation. *Prosthet. Orthot. Int.*, **11**, 113–116.

Weaver, P.C. and Marshall, S.A. (1973) Functional and social review of the lower limb amputee. *Br. J. Surg.*, **60**, 732–737.

3

Conditions leading to amputation

Most amputations are performed for gangrene (from the Greek word gangraina, meaning to gnaw), usually of the lower limb and in men. Gangrene is most often due to vascular disease and the commonest vascular disease is atherosclerosis. Diabetes mellitus is the next commonest cause of gangrene and is often associated with atherosclerosis. These two conditions are the cause of gangrene in 90% of those requiring amputation. Small artery disease, venous disease, trauma, congenital malformations, malignancies and infection make up a very small proportion of the indications for amputation (Table 3.1).

PERIPHERAL VASCULAR DISEASE

Atherosclerosis

Atherosclerosis and its complications account for half of the deaths in the developed world, and it is the commonest reason for amputation. The cause is unknown but there are established risk factors (Table 3.2) and it seems that smoking is the most important potentially reversible cure (Myers et al., 1978; Quick and Cotton, 1982). It is known that reduction of dietary fat and body weight are probably effective although there is still controversy over the cholesterol and triglyceride levels (Greenhalgh, 1984; Shepherd et al., 1987). Control of hypertension is known to diminish the number of strokes. Control of diabetes is obviously desirable but has not been shown to improve the outlook for the patient with peripheral vascular disease. Atherosclerosis is a generalized disease but may affect the limbs, heart or brain separately or together.

Table 3.1 Conditions leading to amputation

1. Peripheral vascular disease		
	Large artery	Atherosclerosis
		Thromboangiitis obliterans
		Thrombosis and embolism
		Trauma
	Small artery	Raynaud's phenomenon
		Arteritis
	Venous	Leg ulcers
2. Diabetes mellitus		
3. Congenital malformation		
4. Malignant disease		
5. Infection		
6. Trauma		

Table 3.2 Risk factors in peripheral atherosclerosis

1. Smoking
2. Diabetes
3. Hypertension
4. Lack of exercise
5. Hyperlipaedaemia
6. Social deprivation (in gangrene)

It is a disease of unknown cause that can affect any part of the arterial system. The basic lesion is the deposition of lipid substances and cholesterol underneath the intimal lining of large and medium-sized arteries (Figure 3.1). This is the atherosclerotic plaque which over a period of years causes fibrosis and narrowing of the affected arteries over a very variable extent (Figure 3.2). Associated with this effect is a fibrosis of the vessel wall that causes so-called 'hardening of the arteries' and in some places a tortuosity commonly seen in the antecubital fossa and in the temporal region. The plaques themselves may cause no trouble, for example in the aorta, but if they affect strategic places then serious sequelae may follow. A single plaque sited at the carotid artery bifurcation (Figure 3.3) may cause cerebral or retinal transient ischaemic attacks, i.e. temporary attacks of paralysis or loss of sensation in the opposite side of the body or blindness on the same side. The carotid plaque ulcerates and liberates emboli of lipid and cholesterol debris into the cerebral circulation causing ischaemia of the cerebral hemisphere or into the retinal arteries causing blindness. These warning attacks may be followed at any time by a permanent stroke. A plaque sited at the origin of a renal artery from the aorta may cause such a narrowing as to lower the blood flow in the affected kidney and produce

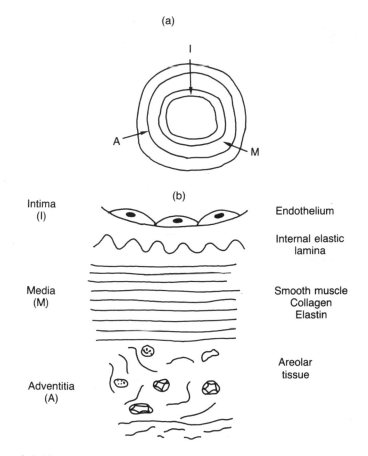

Figure 3.1 Normal arterial wall, transverse section. (a) Macroscopic, (b) microscopic.

renal hypertension. Gangrene of the lower limbs may be due to plaques causing stenosis in one or more leg arteries or the thrombosis that often follows stenosis (Figure 3.2). An artery can be narrowed by as much as 80% of its cross-sectional area before there is a profound fall in blood flow. Once this happens thrombosis may follow of a very variable extent. Gangrene leading to amputation indicates that there is a very severe degree of stenosis or thrombosis, usually in the arteries supplying blood to the legs. The disease in the legs may be mainly proximally sited, aortofemoral, or more often in the femoral artery extending into the popliteal artery, femoropopliteal disease. The lesions are more distally sited less frequently (Figure 3.4). The body has a remarkable

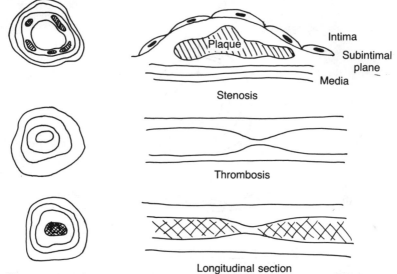

Figure 3.2 Atherosclerosis plaque formation.

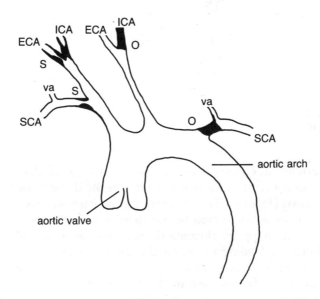

Figure 3.3 Carotid and subclavian artery disease. ECA, external carotid artery; ICA, internal carotid artery, sca, subclavian carotid artery; va, vertebral artery; S, stenosis, O, occlusion (thrombosis).

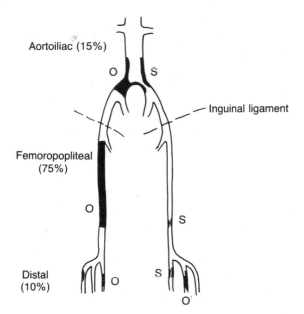

Figure 3.4 Distribution of atherosclerosis in lower limb arteries, S, stenosis, O, occlusion.

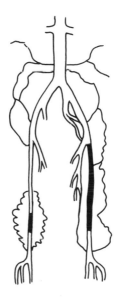

Figure 3.5 Collateral artery development.

capacity to overcome the effects of atherosclerosis and its associated decrease in blood flow by producing collateral vessels (Figure 3.5) that bypass the blocks in the arteries. If these can be produced adequately then there will be no symptoms or signs. If the response is inadequate or the thrombosis is so sudden that the collateral vessels cannot be produced in time then the tissues, usually in toes and feet, may die and gangrene sets in from inadequate perfusion of the tissues with blood. The arms are rarely affected by atherosclerosis, perhaps because the blood pressure in the arm vessels is much lower in the standing position than in the legs and the level of blood pressure may be important in the causation or localization of atherosclerosis; for example, atherosclerosis is seen in the veins only very rarely but can develop when they are implanted into arteries as a bypass to obstruction.

In the abdominal aorta atherosclerosis may predominantly affect the wall from a level just below the origin of the renal arteries (Figure 3.6). Elastic tissue in the aorta is destroyed and dilation or aneurysm formation results under the continuous pressure of the circulating blood. Eventually these aneurysms rupture, usually fatally, 60% within 2 years of their recognition.

Peripheral arterial disease is arterial disease outside the heart. The presentation of atherosclerosis affecting the legs is either as intermittent

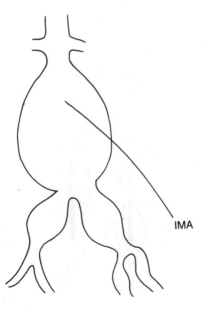

IMA

Figure 3.6 Abdominal aortic aneurysm. IMA, inferior mesenteric artery.

claudication, rest pain or skin colour changes ending with gangrene. Intermittent claudication (Latin claudicare, to limp) is muscular pain coming on after a fixed walking distance and sited in the buttock or thigh (aortoiliac disease) or more often in the calf (aortoiliac or femoro-popliteal disease). The pain forces the subject to stop, then, after a few minutes it goes off, only to return after a similar period of walking. Rest pain is sited in the toes or feet. It is continuous and worse at night when blood flow to the skin is at its lowest due to the fall in cardiac output, pulse rate and blood pressure. Rest pain is serious, representing a severe ischaemia of the skin and nerves whereas claudication is benign due to muscle ischaemia and is relieved by ceasing exercise. Rest pain may go on to be followed by ulceration or gangrene. Colour changes in the extremity may precede gangrene: the skin is dusky, may darken and then blacken as the tissues die. Most patients with gangrene suffer severe pain but if the nerves are destroyed as well as the other tissues in the extremity there will be no pain.

Intermittent claudication

Over the last 40 years, there has been much controversy over therapy for intermittent claudication. This has occurred since studies of the natural history of this symptom have shown the ability of the body to overcome blocks and narrowings of the arterial circulation by the growth of the collateral circulation and so improve the symptoms spontaneously (Jelnes *et al.*, 1986). Approximately 40% of patients presenting with vascular claudication improve spontaneously, 40% are unchanged and 20% need studies possibly leading to reconstructive arterial surgery. Many patients fear gangrene and amputation when they learn they have arterial disease but in fact only 8% require amputation. Claudication can improve spontaneously up to 2 years from its beginning. Telling patients these facts is very therapeutic in that they are reassured that no immediate decision has to be made and if they do deteriorate they can return for assessment. A medical condition in which 80% either improve or do not worsen is not a serious condition. A simple treadmill test establishes the baseline walking distance and arterial blood pressure made by ultrasound measurements at the ankle confirm the diagnosis. Smoking is forbidden and patients are instructed to walk slowly and keep within the limits of their pain. Claudication is known in Germany as 'smoker's legs', (rauchebeine) or the 'shopping window disease' (schaufenster krankheit). Some patients benefit from 'walking training', i.e. supervised exercises under the guidance of a physiotherapist, gradually walking more and more and pushing the patient to the point of pain (Zetterquist, 1970). This is only helpful to those in whom the claudication is of recent onset and the pain-free distance is short. Many patients tolerate their claudication for years and indeed do not appreciate the significance of it, it may even get completely better. Suddenly there may be a sudden deterioration or reappearance of the symptom when presumably a stenosis in an artery has been converted to a thrombosis or a thrombosis may have extended in length and blocked off strategically sited collateral vessels. Patients should be tested for diabetes and have their serum cholesterol and triglyceride levels measured because diabetes is often associated and disturbances of cholesterol and lipid metabolism frequent.

Treadmill testing in 20% of claudicants reveals no evidence of arterial blockage, though pain-free exercise distance is reduced (Blau and Logue, 1957). The usual cause of 'pseudoclaudication' arises from back trouble, prolapsed intervertebral disc, osteoarthritis or spinal stenosis with or without neurological signs and symptoms. Most patients have had some back complaints previously. Because peripheral vascular disease and spinal disease are both common, the two often coexist making assessment of the contribution of each condition very difficult even after ultrasonography, angiography, radiculography and computerized tomography.

There have been many therapeutic trials for intermittent claudication over the years. Lumbar sympathectomy was a favoured operation performed to denervate the muscle arterioles and possibly improve blood flow. Many studies showed a 40% success rate which of course is well within the spontaneous relief rate. Muscle arterioles are dilated by the accumulation of metabolites which are already maximal in ischaemic muscle and finally, there are few or no vasoconstrictor fibres in skeletal muscle. For all these reasons lumbar sympathectomy is no longer performed for intermittent claudication. Other historical operations have been performed to limit walking distance, for example section of nerves to the calf muscle and section of the tendo calcaneum.

Innumerable drugs have been used for pain due to vascular disease (Table 3.3) and a glance at MIMS, the pharmaceutical trade dictionary of drugs, shows 20 or more medicines used in peripheral vascular disease but it must be admitted that none has been conclusively proven to be more effective than natural improvement (Clyne, 1980). The most common group used are the peripheral arterial dilators which act either by direct effect on the vessel wall or by blocking the sympathetic vasoconstriction activity. There is no doubt that these drugs are effective in normal vessels, in animals or by intravenous or intra-arterial injection but their effect in atherosclerotic patients is only transient, or

Table 3.3 Drugs for vascular disease – modes of action

Proprietary name	Registered name	Primary 'vascular' action	Other effects
Isoxsuprine	Duvadilan Defencin	β-adrenergic blockers	β-adrenergic stimulant
Cyclandelate	Cyclospasmol Cyclobral		β-adrenergic stimulant
Thymoxamine	Opilon		
Phenoxybenzamine	Dibenyline		
Tolazoline	Priscol		
Nicotinic acid (and related substances)	Hexopal Bradilan Ronicol Vasculit	Direct effects on vessel wall	Effects on lipid metabolism
Bamethan		Effects on lipid metabol sm	
Nicotinic acid (and related substances)	Hexopal Bradilan Ronicol		
Vasolastine	Vasolastine Atromid-S		
Clofibrate			Reduces serum fibrinogen
Oxpentifylline	Trental	Effects on blood viscosity	
Cinnarizine	Stugeron		Antihistamine and labyrinth depressant
Naftidrofuryl	Praxilene	Effects on muscle metabolism	

ineffective. Vitamin E acts as an antioxidant and eliminates free radicals that may be harmful to tissues. Hypoglycaemic agents were tried because of anecdotal reports of claudication improving in diabetic patients treated with orally administered hypoglycaemic agents. Both alpha and beta ganglion blocking agents act on sympathetic nerve transmitters at the level of the sympathetic ganglia. In fact some patients treated for hypertension with beta blocking agents find their peripheral ischaemic symptoms become worse. Metabolic stimulants are said to act by improving the uptake of oxygen by the tissues. Many patients with vascular disease have a higher blood viscosity level than normal due partly to raised fibrinogen levels or to an increased blood red cell mass. Smoking is associated with a relative polycythaemia and hence a raised viscosity (Lowe *et al.*, 1981). Recent studies have shown significant improvements in the mortality of heart attacks using viscosity reducing drugs but no studies have yet been produced of improvements in the symptoms of peripheral vascular disease. Red cells 7 µm in diameter have to pass through capillaries 3–5 µm in diameter, and therefore have to be very flexible. In arterial disease and many other conditions the red cell membrane becomes more rigid than normal. There are drugs that can increase red cell flexibility. Serotonin is a substance liberated from platelets that can cause local vasospasm. Serotonin antagonists are claimed to be effective for most ischaemic symptoms produced in both large and small vessel disease. Calcium channel blocking agents are effective in angina pectoris but have not been shown to be effective in intermittent claudication. Prostanoids, derivatives of naturally occurring prostacyclin, are potent vasodilators and platelet disaggregators. Intravenously administered, they dramatically produce flushing and hypotension but their role in arterial disease is probably going to be limited to small vessel disease.

Arterial reconstruction by dilatation, rebore or bypass, is the most dramatically successful treatment for intermittent claudication for it restores the arterial inflow into the muscles, in many cases completely. These procedures are, however, often major operations which have complications and mortality, especially as they are performed on older people with associated coronary and cerebral atherosclerosis or other smoking-related diseases, such as bronchitis, emphysema and even cancer of the lung. They are more successful when the disease is sited above the inguinal ligament where the arteries are large and blood flow is high. Because so many patients with intermittent claudication improve spontaneously over a long period of time and their symptoms are relieved by inactivity most surgeons are reluctant to operate for claudication alone. If, however, the pain-free distance is decreasing and if it falls below 100 m or if it is associated with rest pain, coldness or numbness, then an operation must be seriously considered. Now that balloon dilatation (percutaneous transluminal angioplasty) of stenosis and limited occlusion is established, this manoeuvre carried out by the interventional radiologist, has widened the indication for relatively non-invasive treatment, especially for less severe claudication due to disease in the aortoiliac segment. The results are not so good in the femoral artery where the effectiveness is about 65% over 3 years. It is a matter of judgement as to the selection of cases but it has certainly led to a greater use of angiography and certainly angiography of the non-invasive type, such as transvenous digital subtraction angiography. Further developments will probably depend on the use of a laser beam to vaporize occlusions with or without the assistance of balloon angioplasty.

Rest pain

Rest pain is a serious symptom and in many cases a warning of the onset of gangrene. It is agonizing and in many cases only relieved by opiates, arterial reconstruction, or amputation. All cases merit immediate admission into hospital for consideration of operation. On admission diabetes and hypertension are controlled and anaemia, if present, corrected. If there is any infection in the foot or toes this is treated with antibiotics. With this regimen and rest a few patients, about one in ten, do get spontaneous relief. Sympathectomy (Cotton and Cross, 1985; Campbell, 1988) (chemical) has an important role in pain relief in about half of cases; the rest go on to angiography with a view to possible arterial reconstruction. In some cases nothing positive can be done and amputation is the only way forward. The use of intravenous drugs, vasodilators and metabolic stimulants has not been proven of value, except perhaps in relieving pain for a short period previous to operation.

Gangrene

Gangrenous areas are areas of dead tissue which must be removed by operation or less often by spontaneous separation through the line of demarcation that marks the junction of living and dead tissues. Gangrene may be minimal, involving only the tips of digits, as seen in Raynaud's phenomenon, where small vessels are involved, for example digital arteries. More extensive gangrene involving whole digits and extending into the forefoot suggests that larger vessels are occluded or narrowed from the tibial to iliac vessels. Sudden onset suggests a sudden change in arteries such as thrombosis or embolism. 'Venous gangrene' is the result of massive occlusion of veins both major and minor with or without arterial occlusion. Gangrene should be kept as dry as possible, wet gangrene implies an infection that can spread locally and by blood. The extremities should be kept horizontal. Dependency which may give some relief is harmful because of the accumulation of tissue fluid due to failure of the calf muscle pump to clear blood efficiently from the dependent lower limb. Culture of gangrenous areas usually grows a mixture of saprophytic organisms and pathogens, aerobic and anaerobic. *Staphylococci* and gas-forming anaerobes are always worrying, not only because of what they do to the patient but also because they provide a focus of cross-infection in a ward. Such cases are, if possible, best isolated and given appropriate antibiotics. The diagnosis of gas gangrene is clinical and radiological. The mere presence of anaerobes in an area of gangrene does not necessarily indicate the clinical diagnosis of gas gangrene which implies an infection of muscle with gas-forming organisms.

Examination and investigation

A general clinical assessment is made by the history and physical signs. Disorders such as diabetes and hypertension and smoking-related diseases such as bronchitis, emphysema and carcinoma of the lung are looked for. Cardiac problems such as angina pectoris, arrhythmias and bradycardia are common. Blood disorders may be related; polycythaemia (increased red cell mass) and thrombocythaemia (increase in platelets) occur and anaemia is common from blood loss or poor nutrition. Renal function may be poor, often due to prostatism. Basic tests required are blood count, blood grouping and cross-matching if an operation is indicated, and urine testing for glucose and albumen. Blood is taken for measurement of urea, creatinine and electrolytes. Chest radiographs and electrocardiographs are essential, if only as a baseline for the possibility of future changes, especially after surgery.

The clinical history indicates the presence of arterial disease and the physical signs indicate its localization. Peripheral pulses are carefully palpated and both sides compared for differences in pulse amplitude. Bruits heard over the groin indicate the presence of disease-causing stenosis in the aortoiliac segment. Silence over an absent femoral pulse indicates a complete occlusion proximally, a noise indicates stenosis. Coldness, unless extreme, is of no import as the covering of clothes may well warm up an ischaemic limb; skin colour changes should be recorded.

Treadmill testing is useful for measuring the pain-free walking distance of claudicants because most patients find it impossible to give an accurate figure of how many yards or metres they can walk. A distance of less than 100 m is serious if it is maintained at that level for some weeks or months. Many patients with rest pain or gangrene do not have claudication, either because they cannot walk or because the ischaemia is of skin rather than of muscles due to the pattern of vascular occlusion. For example, where the disease is affecting the tibial arteries alone or in association with more proximal occlusion in the femoro-popliteal or aortoiliac segments, reconstruction of these proximal occlusions or stenoses may overcome the more distally sited disease, relieve rest pain and avoid the need for amputation.

Measurement of the pressure index by Doppler insonation is useful in gauging the severity of the disease and in some cases its localization (Bernstein, 1982; Goss et al., 1988). The Doppler probe enables the examiner to measure blood pressure of the extremities in recumbency. Normally blood pressure at the ankle is the same as in the brachial or slightly higher in some cases due to artefact. A lower pressure at the ankle than the brachial indicates a blockage in the arterial tree proximally. The ratio of pedal to brachial pressure is the pressure index (PI), normally one or greater than one. In claudicants the PI is usually less than 0.8, in rest pain less than 0.6, and below 0.4 gangrene is likely.

The pulse wave-form can be printed from the signal obtained from a bidirectional Doppler probe and can be analysed by many mathematical procedures. It had been hoped that such an analysis of the femoral flow wave-form might be of value in detecting the presence of aortoiliac disease but this has not been proven.

Percutaneous transfemoral puncture is the usual route of radiological evaluation of the peripheral arterial tree. A flexible catheter is inserted into the femoral artery over a guide wire which is removed and the catheter advanced to lie just below the renal arteries. Rapid injection of radiopaque medium allows radiological exposures to be made of the whole arterial tree from the abdominal aorta to the pedal arches of the feet. Where a catheter cannot be passed because of the lack of femoral pulsation then a translumbar approach is required through a needle inserted into the aorta from the left side with the patient prone. Intravenous digital subtraction angiology is a less invasive method of radiological investigation. The contrast medium is given intravenously and it can be performed as an out-patient manoeuvre and repeated often. It is especially useful in carotid artery examination and for follow-up studies of arterial reconstruction looking for faults and complications that can be anticipated rather than having to wait for their full and possibly catastrophic effect on the limb.

Sophisticated ultrasonic imaging can be used to give images of blood vessels and measure blood flow. This is a totally non-invasive investigation and very useful for the diagnosis of carotid artery disease. Arteries can also be visualized by nuclear magnetic resonance. The machines used for the above procedures are all expensive and are found in relatively few centres. The minimum need is for aortography and next for digital subtraction angiography.

THROMBOANGIITIS OBLITERANS (BUERGER'S DISEASE)

This is a rare form of arterial disease that many surgeons regard as a variant of atherosclerosis in young individuals. Most presenting atherosclerotic patients are over the age of 50 or 60 years but there is a group of patients who present with ischaemic symptoms at a much younger age, usually in their twenties or thirties or even their teens. The distinctive features are a younger age of onset, men are affected almost exclusively, heavy smoking is universal, the disease is usually peripherally sited, affecting medium-sized arteries such as the tibial arteries and beyond.

Pathological examination in the early stages of the disease may suggest an inflammatory process involving the whole vascular bundle, arteries, veins and nerves. The cause is often of long duration, extending over many years with long periods of apparent remission. It is a rare condition but undoubtedly does occur and it may be a manifestation of other types of arteritis which are even more rare. In extreme cases all four limbs are affected, and it is commonly complicated by heart disease and strokes.

ARTERIAL EMBOLISM AND ACUTE THROMBOSIS

An embolus is a foreign body in the circulation, that may be due to fat from broken bones after a severe injury, amniotic fluid after child birth or a foreign body such as a bullet which has entered the circulation or migrated into it. The radiologist may inject emboli of foreign material to block off vessels, for example in young children with arteriovenous malformations, or to shrink down a tumour such as in the kidney. However, the commonest arterial embolus is a thrombus coming from

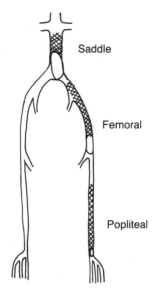

Figure 3.7 Arterial embolism.

the heart, usually from the left auricle when it is fibrillating or from the left ventricle after a myocardial infarction. The usual cardiac disease is mitral stenosis which leads to a buildup of thrombus in the left atrium. When the atrium fibrillates it is prone to liberate thrombi into the arterial tree, which may result in death of tissue by infarction. If an embolus gets into the cerebral circulation a stroke may result, splenic or renal infarcts may be caused, and in the superior mesenteric artery fatal gangrene of the gut is likely. More often emboli occur in the peripheral arteries of both upper and lower limbs; usually they lodge at bifurcations where the divided arteries are naturally smaller (Figure 3.7). An embolus at the aortic bifurcation causes ischaemia of the legs, at the femoral bifurcation below the groin one leg is affected. Many emboli cause ischaemic symptoms that improve spontaneously due to slippage of the embolus into less important vessels or the development of an adequate collateral supply, but in most cases the embolus must be removed surgically and as soon as possible, for beyond the site of lodgement thrombus forms which blocks up progressively more and more of the distal arterial circulation and hence the possibility of its efficient removal is reduced. Acute arterial thrombosis may simulate arterial embolism, although usually there are previous existing symptoms of arterial disease such as intermittent claudication (see p.29). It may be treated as embolism by removal of the thrombus but it is likely that thrombosis will recur because of the underlying disease. Thrombolytic therapy and balloon angioplasty may be indicated.

RAYNAUD'S PHENOMENON

Vascular disease affecting major arteries and causing gangrene that can only be treated by amputation in most cases leads to a major amputation, usually of the leg either above or below the knee. Vascular disease affecting small arteries when it is severe may cause digital gangrene more often in the hands than in the feet which may lead to minor amputation of parts or the whole of digits. Raynaud's phenomenon, described first by Maurice Raynaud in 1862, is a clinical phenomenon manifested by cold sensitivity. In this condition fingers and toes go white and are painful on exposure to cold, go red when they are warmed up or quite often the extremities are purply blue (acrocyanosis). The whiteness is due to small vessel spasm, the redness to reactive hyperaemia after an episode of spasm and the blueness due to oxygen-poor blood in the cutaneous venules. Every degree of severity is experienced. In the most extreme cases gangrene or ulcers, usually of tips of fingers, may appear which are painful and cause discharge. Not many of these patients require surgery but when they do it is usually limited to drainage of abscesses and removal of gangrenous tips of fingers or toes and much more rarely amputation of digit. The gangrene rarely extends more proximally than the metacarpophalangeal joint.

VENOUS ULCERS

Ulcers of the leg due to venous disease, varicose veins or the results of deep vein thrombosis are common, an incidence of 150 000 in the UK has been quoted (Figure 3.8). Venous disease causes failure of the calf muscle pump to clear the blood from the leg because of damage to the veins or valves in them, unlike arterial disease where the failure is to get enough arterial blood to the legs because of arterial occlusion or narrowing. Failure to clear blood from the legs results in waterlogging of the tissues and ulceration which is relieved by recumbency or pressure bandaging of the legs. Most cases of ulcers can be healed by pressure bandaging and, if possible, dealing with associated varicose veins by surgical operation. Some ulcers become chronic, and many encircle the lower leg and cause much misery, pain and discharge. Even more rarely

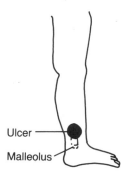

Figure 3.8 Venous ulcer.

malignancy, in the form of a squamous cell carcinoma, may arise in the ulcer, usually after many years (Marjolin's ulcer). Amputation may then be indicated, usually below the knee. Local lymph nodes in the groin may increase in size. Cases are rare and subjects affected are usually very old.

DIABETES MELLITUS

Foot problems are very common in patients afflicted by diabetes mellitus. The three important predisposing factors are infection, neuropathy and atherosclerosis. Diabetics are very susceptible to bacterial infection so that what would be a trivial infection in a non-diabetic can become very serious in a diabetic. Peripheral neuropathy is common in diabetes, particularly in the legs and feet. In this condition there is a degeneration of the peripheral nerves, leading to loss of sensory and proprioceptive sensation in the foot and ankle, that in turn leads to numbness. There may be loss of ankle reflexes and joint sensation and vibration sense. Occasionally the condition is extremely painful. The small muscles of the foot atrophy and lead to deformities of the toes and feet, such as clawed toes and dropped arches. The sensory loss is often associated with perforating ulcers, particularly on the under surface of the metatarsophalangeal joint of the great toe. These ulcers are usually insensitive. Joints may become disorganized (Charcot joints). Gangrene is a common complication; in some cases the microcirculation in the affected areas is changed dramatically. Degeneration may damage the sympathetic nervous supply to the arterioles, leading to a hot dry foot – autosympathectomy. There is evidence also of open communications between small arteries and veins (arteriovenous anastomoses) so that pulses may be bounding and arterial blood flow in a leg higher than normal and yet there are areas of peripheral gangrene. Such gangrenous and infected areas usually heal well with drainage of abscesses and local removal of dead tissue. Many atherosclerotic patients (20–40%) have known or latent evidence of diabetes, more often of the non-insulin-dependent type. The contribution of each of these factors – infection, neuropathy and atherosclerosis – is variable and so the likelihood of healing or amputation is difficult to predict and is usually a matter of trial. Where small arteries are affected, clearing up infection and local removal of dead tissue often results in healing.

TRAUMA

Amputation following trauma can be an immediate or delayed procedure and is necessary for any of the following reasons: extensive tissue destruction, vascular impairment, neurological damage, burns and bony non-union. Amputation should not represent therapeutic failure and the proper role of amputation should be defined (Lange, 1989). The main causes of amputation in the west are road traffic, farming and industrial accidents. In other parts of the world the main cause is warfare. The numbers of amputations following trauma in the UK are falling as practice at the worksite becomes safer (Ham et al., 1989). Occasionally amputations are necessary for cases of osteomyelitis arising after a fracture, or after poliomyelitis where the muscle is so damaged as to make the link useless.

Early amputation is necessary where the limb is ischaemic, the nerve supply severed or there has been a loss of skin, muscle or bone. All viable tissue should be conserved at the initial operation. Cleaning and removal of the dead tissue is necessary followed by a guillotine amputation. Resuturing takes place approximately 5 days later when the risk of infection has fallen and the wound site is clean. As much bone length and skin as possible is kept to enable as many surgical options as possible to be considered at a later time.

Amputations at a later time generally take place when the tissues are non-viable or gangrene is present. Following extensive damage, the amputation may take place later when other damage is identified, for example articular damage, extensive skin loss and functional loss. Amputations may also take place years following an accident for reasons of bony nonunion, pain or disability.

The decision to amputate is a multifactorial clinical decision but this should be made as early as possible. Often the decision has to be delayed until after medicolegal outcomes are resolved and the true symptoms are identified. Each individual case must be thoroughly assessed medically, functionally, socially and vocationally.

In most cases where large vessels are injured surgical reconstruction is possible. Limbs or parts of limbs can be reimplanted with success so long as the affected part is preserved, cooled and replaced as early as possible. Severe crushing injuries where tissues are widely damaged are the usual indication for amputation in trauma or where arteries are too small or perhaps diseased with atherosclerosis to allow reconstruction, for example in the leg below the knee. Another indication may be failure after arterial reconstruction following an injury.

CONGENITAL MALFORMATIONS

There are 100 per 100 000 children born with a major deformity in the west and the majority of these are of the upper limb (63%). The lower limb accounts for 19% and both upper and lower limbs 18% (Vitali *et al.*, 1986). The deformity is either a failure of formation, differentiation or duplication and leads to overgrowth, undergrowth or general skeletal abnormalities. The cause is varied, ranging from a congenital band *in utero*, drug-induced thalidomide, familial or from unknown factors.

Babies may be born with limbs so grossly deformed that amputation can only be offered in the hope of a normal development with a prosthesis. Some cases are associated with neurofibromatosis, others are a result of the thalidomide tragedy. More common is deformity from a vascular malformation that may lead to overdevelopment or less often underdevelopment of a limb, usually associated with a birth mark of the plane variety that may cover part or the whole of the skin of a limb. Early on, this is livid in colour but often pales off over a period of years leaving a coppery tinge. There is a wide spectrum of vascular anomalies. At one end of the spectrum only the veins are affected, as varicose veins or swelling of the leg appearing in childhood often with some increased length of the limb or a large foot. At the other end of the spectrum there is gross evidence of arteriovenous shunting (Figure 3.9). The limb is hot, flushed, with bounding pulses and even pulsating veins. The whole limb or just digits or part of the limb is greatly overdeveloped both in length and in girth, fingers or toes may be grossly enlarged. The volume of the left to right arterial shunt may impose a burden on the heart and there is a risk of irreversible left ventricular failure. Most cases are treated by the radiologists who embolize the shunts through a catheter inserted

41

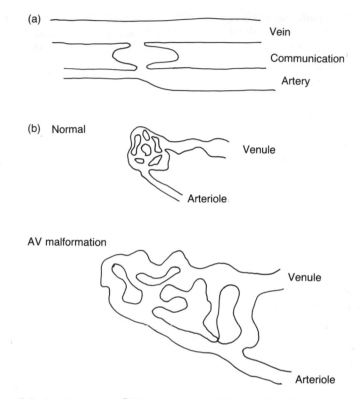

Figure 3.9 Arteriovenous CAV aneurysm. (a) Traumatic, (b) congenital.

into a strategically sited artery for feeding. Many substances have been used, one is gelatine sponge which can be injected through a needle and forms a plug in the affected area. Occasionally in localized malformations and where there is extensive involvement of bone or where embolization has failed, amputation may become inevitable and may be curative.

Recording of the deficiency has now been standardized and is either total, partial and described as either a transverse or longitudinal plane (see International Standard 8548).

MALIGNANT DISEASE

Amputations for malignancy account for a small percentage of amputees in the UK (Ham *et al.*, 1989). The most common primary malignant tumour is osteosarcoma. This generally occurs in young patients in the second decade of life in the femur, tibia or humerus. The distal femur and upper tibia are the most commonly affected (Balsam, 1980). The symptoms include bone pain, swelling and a limp and the rate of growth of the tumour and its blood-borne dissemination to the lungs give a poor prognosis. Survival rates of between 12 and 20% at 5 years of age are reported (Weiss *et al.*, 1978; Kingston, personnal communication, 1990). The longer survival rates occur where the tumour is in the distal end of the bone. The current practice is to treat the lesion for 3–4 months by radiotherapy and then amputate if no metastases are seen radiologically and on isotopic computerized scanning. Patients who had surgery and chemotherapy lived one and a half months longer than those who had surgery alone (Weiss *et al.*, 1978). The chemotherapy shrinks the tumour and it is used to help prevent metastases. The side effects are: temporary hair loss, nausea, vomiting, renal toxity, hearing loss or loss of high tones and cardiotoxicity.

The second most common primary malignant tumours are the chondrosarcoma and Ewing's sarcoma. These tumours are usually seen in the 30–50 year age group and they affect the long bones, pelvis and ribs. They are slow-growing tumours and remain locally invasive for many years. The majority of hindquarter amputations are performed for chondrosarcoma. Ewing's sarcoma occurs at a wider range of age and the symptoms include bone pain, swelling, pain, malaise and weight loss.

Amputation may occasionally be necessary for malignant melanoma, particularly on the legs or arms. Squamous, basal cell, soft tissue tumour, fibrosarcoma, neurofibrosarcoma and visceral cancers involving the bladder, uterus and rectum do occasionally lead to amputation. Malignant tumours which are secondary lesions are more common in the limbs than primary lesions, generally spreading from primary tumours of the breast, prostate, lung, thyroid, kidney and the adrenal cortex. Some of these tumours today respond to radiotherapy, chemotherapy or hormonal agents but secondary renal carcinoma is the one most likely to lead to amputation if radiotherapy and chemotherapy fail.

It used to be said that amputation should be carried out at a level one joint above the site of the tumour but as many of them are in the femur this would mean disarticulation of the hip. Today most amputations are performed in the thigh but this naturally depends upon the location of the tumour growth. Most soft tissue sarcomas can be excised locally unless bone is involved.

INFECTION

Gas gangrene is an infection that may necessitate amputation. It is common in warfare where wounds are likely to be contaminated with soil in which anaerobic organisms can grow. This is a problem of war and is rarely encountered in peace time. The principles of treatment are wound toilet, drainage, chemotherapy and leaving wounds open rather than closed, very rarely may amputation be necessary as an emergency. Hyperbaric oxygen has been used but has little place now. Gas gangrene is a real possibility after amputation of a leg, from contamination of the amputation stump from the patient's faecal organisms in the presence of ischaemic tissue and often in diabetics. For this reason all amputees should be given antibiotics for aerobic and anaerobic organisms in the post-operative period. Gas gangrene is still highly fatal. Infection is suspected if the patient is unwell, febrile and showing tachycardia. The wound should be inspected for the typical coppery discolouring of skin and the typical fetid smell.

Bubbles of gas may appear in the wound discharge or be felt in the subcutaneous tissues as crepitus around the wound or show up as gas bubbles in X-rays of the stump. Chronic infection leading to amputation is rare but may be necessary if there is a chronic osteomyelitis due to an unresolved infection or perhaps after injury or after involvement by malignant disease.

REFERENCES

Balsam, F.J. (1980) Rehabilitation of the lower extremity cancer amputee. *MD Stat. Med. J.*, **29**, 85–87.

Bernstein, E.E. (1982) *Noninvasive Diagnostic Techniques in Vascular Disease*. C.V. Mosby, St Louis.

Blau, I.N. and Logue, V. (1957) Intermittent claudication of the cauda equina. *Lancet*, **i**, 1081.

Campbell, W.B. (1988) Sympathectomy for chronic arterial ischaemia. *Eur. J. Vasc. Surg.*, **2**, 357.

Clyne, C.A.C. (1980) Non-surgical management of peripheral vascular disease: a review. *Br. Med. J.*, **281**, 794.

Cotton, L.T. and Cross, F.W. (1985) Lumbar sympathectomy for arterial disease. *Br. J. Surg.*, **72**, 678.

Goss, D.E., Simpson, J., Roberts, V.C. and Cotton, L.T. (1988) Evaluation of a computerised test for the assessment of peripheral vascular disease. *Eur. Vasc. Surg.*, **2**, 333.

Greenhalgh, R.M. (1984) Management of risk factors in patients undergoing arterial surgery, in *Arterial Surgery (Clinical Surgery 8)* (ed. J.J. Bergan), Churchill Livingstone, Edinburgh.

Ham, R.O., Luff, R. and Roberts, V.C. (1989) A five year review for prosthetic treatment in England, Wales and Northern Ireland 1981–1985. *Health Trends*, **21**, 3–6.

Jelnes, R., Gaardsting, O., Hougaard, X., Jensen, K., Baekgard, N., Tonnesen, K.H. and Schroeder, T. (1986) Fate in intermittent claudication: outcome and risks. *Br. Med. J.*, **293**, 1137.

Lange, R.H. (1989) Limb reconstruction versus amputation. Decision making in massive lower extremity trauma. *Clin. Orth. Rel. Res.*, **243**, 92–99.

Lowe, G.D.O., Barbenel, J.C. and Forbes, C.D. (1981) *Clinical Aspects of Blood Viscosity and Cell Deformity*. Springer-Verlag, Berlin.

Myers, K.A., King, R.B. and Scott, N. (1978) The effect of smoking on the late patency of arterial reconstructions on the legs. *Br. J. Surg.*, **65**, 267.

Quick, C.R.G. and Cotton, L.T. (1982) The measured effect of stopping smoking on intermittent claudication. *Br. J. Surg.*, **69** (Suppl.), 24.

Shepherd, J., Betteridge, D.J., Durrington, P., Laker, M., Lewis, B., Mann, J., Miller, J.P., Reckless, J.P.D. and Thompson, S.R. (1987) Strategies for reducing coronary heart disease and desirable limits for blood lipid concentrations: guidelines of the British Hyperlipaedaemia Association. *Br. Med. J.*, **295**, 1245.

Vitali, M., Robinson, K.P., Harris, E.E. and Redhead, R.G. (1986) Management of congenital deformities, in *Amputations and Prostheses*, Baillière Tindall, London, pp. 202–212.

Weiss, A.B., Adams, G., Brackin, B., Pritchett, P. and Moreno, H. (1978) Osteosarcoma. *Clin. Orth. Rel. Res.*, **135**, 137–147.

Zetterquist, S. (1970) The effect of active training on the nutritive blood flow in exercising ischaemic legs. *Scand. J. Clin. Im. Lab. Inv.*, **25**, 102.

4

Operations for the relief of arterial disease

The operations used in the relief of arterial disorders are lumbar sympathectomy, arterial reconstruction, balloon angioplasty and amputation.

LUMBAR SYMPATHECTOMY

The thoracolumbar outflow of the sympathetic nervous system leaves the spinal cord at the level of the first thoracic segment down to the second or third lumbar segment (Figure 4.1). The sympathetic ganglia are arranged segmentally; in the chest they lie on the neck of the ribs and in the lumbar region on the transverse processes of the lumbar vertebrae. From the ganglia they travel with the nerve plexuses and on the way down the limbs give off branches to adjacent vessels, arteries and veins, until the final arterial branches innervate the arterioles. Dilatation and constriction of arterioles very much control the blood flow to the capillaries and hence to the tissues. In arterial disease, particularly in cases of rest pain, the affected parts are the toes and feet which are innervated in the area of the dermatomes lumbar four and five and sacral one and two (Figure 4.2).

The sympathetic outflow for these dermatomes in the spinal cord must therefore ascend the cord to come out through the sympathetic outflow of the ganglion at lumbar two ganglion level and then pass down the ganglionated cord to reach the appropriate ganglion. It is usual in sympathectomy to ablate the second and third lumbar ganglia partly because of the safety of access, for L1 ganglion lies behind the renal artery and L4 lies behind the common iliac artery. The second and third lumbar ganglia are isolated and removed in operative sympathectomy.

In chemical sympathectomy the patient is sat up and needles inserted

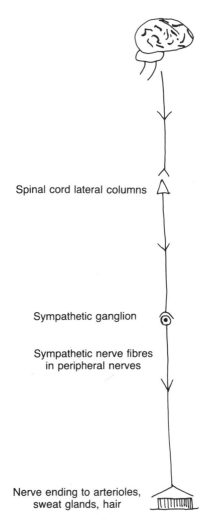

Spinal cord lateral columns

Sympathetic ganglion

Sympathetic nerve fibres
in peripheral nerves

Nerve ending to arterioles,
sweat glands, hair

Figure 4.1 Sympathetic nervous system.

that pass between the transverse processes of the second, third and fourth lumbar vertebrae into the psoas muscle where their position is checked by radiology. A solution of 8% phenol in glycerol is injected around the site of the L2 and L3 lumbar sympathetic ganglia. Phenol is toxic to tissues and will destroy them, glycerol keeps the phenol from spreading and prolongs its effect.

Operative sympathectomy requires a general anaesthetic and is a major performance for the sort of patient who has severe arterial

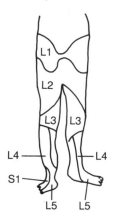

Figure 4.2 Dermatomes lower limb.

disease. It carries both a mortality and morbidity as in any operation in the old, leading to cardiac, pulmonary, bladder, cerebral and infectious complications. Chemical sympathectomy can be an out-patient procedure. It has no mortality, numbness and pain in the area of supply of the lateral cutaneous nerve (L1) over the outer upper thigh occurs in 20% of subjects but usually only persists over a period of weeks or months. This is a procedure for the expert who is usually an anaesthetist experienced in pain relief. Only about 60% of sympathectomies are effective so many operations are of no avail. If a chemical sympathectomy fails there is little lost. The pressure index is helpful, below 0.2 sympathectomy is ineffective. Insulin-dependent diabetics often do not improve.

In the young patient with thromboangiitis obliterans, for example, the effect of a lumbar sympathectomy is often obvious, a warm dry limb with distended superficial veins (the veins are denervated as well as the arteries). In older patents few of these signs may be present although usually the veins are distended to some extent. However, many patients are better with sympathectomy, particularly those with rest pain and minimal gangrene. It should not be used for claudicants or those with more extensive gangrene.

ARTERIAL RECONSTRUCTION

Arterial reconstruction is by bypass, patch graft or balloon angioplasty. It has a relatively short history, dating from the Korean War in 1951 when it was realized that a soldier with an arterial wound could be flown by helicopter virtually from the front line within minutes of wounding to a fully equipped base hospital perhaps a hundred miles away where an arterial reconstruction could be carried out with a great hope of success instead of amputation. Some arterial repairs were performed in the First and Second World Wars but most failed because of the lateness of operations and infection of wounds. During the Second World War there was greater knowledge, antibiotics and blood transfusions but it was speed of transport that really made arterial surgery practicable for trauma. It was the development of the plastic arterial prosthesis that opened the way to widespread arterial reconstruction. Originally arterial reconstruction was more or less limited to rebore or bypass. Rebore was for limited arterial stenosis and occlusion and is still used for carotid artery stenosis. Bypass was for long obstructions or aneurysms. More and more rebore has been replaced by angioplasty using a balloon to overcome an arterial reconstruction, a radiological procedure or a plastic patch to widen an artery permanently by surgical operation. Arterial reconstruction for atherosclerosis in the legs is more successful in the larger arteries above the level of the inguinal ligament, i.e. the aorta and iliac arteries. Below the level of the inguinal ligament where the arteries are small in diameter the failure rate is greater, partly due to the size of the vessels and the diffuse nature of the disease. The 'run in' from the iliac arteries must be unimpeded and the 'run off' not too depleted for success.

AORTOFEMORAL BYPASS

There are many types of plastic prosthesis (Skotnicki *et al.*, 1985) but they can be divided into four categories depending on the type of plastic used: Dacron or Teflon and the weave, knitted or woven. Prostheses may be inserted as straight grafts or bifurcated grafts (trouser grafts). Straight grafts are used for aortic aneurysm replacement where the dilatation does not extend into the iliac arteries. Most aneurysms can be replaced by grafts inserted within the abdomen. Atherosclerotic obstruction is much more extensive and needs a bifurcated graft inserted into the femoral arteries between the inguinal ligament below and the aorta above (Figure 4.3). The type of graft used depends very much on the surgeon's personal preference. The ideal graft should provoke no tissue reaction because this might lead to graft failure or infection and yet should be incorporated into the body's tissues which is ultimately a contradiction in terms.

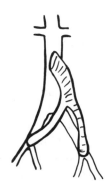

Figure 4.3 Aortoiliac (trouser) graft.

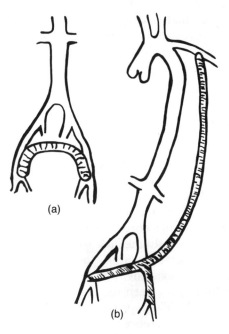

Figure 4.4 Extra-anatomical grafts. (a) Crossover femorofemoral, (b) axillo-bifemoral.

The graft is well incorporated at each end where it is sutured to the host vessels by an extension of the patient's own intima growing over the suture line to a variable extent along the graft. Most of the graft is lined by a 'pseudo intima' deposited from the circulating blood and formed of fibrinogen and platelets. It was felt that lifting up the parts of the new intima and pseudointima might cause thrombosis in the graft. Knitted prostheses were next produced with interstices in the weave large enough to allow macrophages and fibroblasts to grow from outside into the intima and thus fix it. Knitted grafts have to be pre-clotted with the patient's own blood so that the interstices are full of fibrin and clot otherwise devastating blood loss would follow. Experience over the years has shown little difference between the different grafts in terms of their long-term patency and more and more woven grafts are being used. Where there are double lesions in both the aortoiliac and femoropopliteal segments relief of obstruction in the more proximal aortoiliac region often produces enough benefit to avoid a second operation on the distal segment.

Extra-anatomical grafts (Figure 4.4) are used most commonly in patients who are unfit for a major operation such as an aortofemoral bypass and yet there is gangrene due wholly or in part to obstruction in the aortofemoral segment. Other extra-anatomical grafts are employed to bypass sepsis. For example, an infected graft in the groin can be bypassed from the common iliac artery within the pelvis and then passed through the obturator foramen to be joined with the femoral artery at mid-thigh level. Extra-anatomical grafts are not as successful as the aortofemoral bypass. They are often performed either for people too hold or unfit for major surgery or to bypass severe sepsis. Crossover femorofemoral grafts function best.

The axillofemoral graft is a long straight graft, usually 8 mm in diameter, inserted between the axillary artery in the armpit and one or both common femoral arteries in the groin through a tunnel deep through the pectoral muscles and the abdominal skin. Because the graft may easily be compressed where it lies subcutaneously in the flank the lower part of the graft may be strengthened by rings of reinforcing plastic (Kenney et al., 1982). If both legs are affected the graft may be bifurcated or an oblique limb may be sutured to the main graft at one end and to the common femoral artery at the other through a channel where it runs subcutaneously or under the rectus muscle sheath.

The most common extra-anatomical graft is the femorofemoral graft used when one common iliac artery is blocked or when one limb of a trouser graft is blocked. A crossover graft is employed connecting both common femoral arteries running either subcutaneously or deep to the rectus muscles.

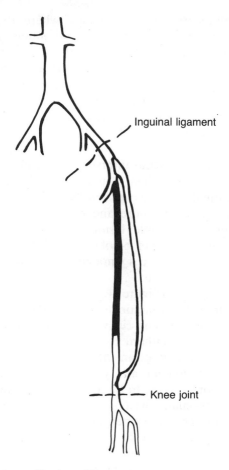

Figure 4.5 Femoropopliteal graft.

FEMOROPOPLITEAL BYPASS

Femoropopliteal disease is a much more common cause of gangrene than aortoiliac disease (Figure 4.5). Although many types of grafts have been used the best is still the patient's own long saphenous vein anastomosed above to the common femoral artery and below preferably to the popliteal artery above the level of the knee joint, though the extent of disease may indicate an infragenicular anastomosis. The graft may be inserted *in situ* in which case its valves must be destroyed with special cutters or scissors and all significant tributaries tied off or these will form sites of arteriovenous communication. More commonly the vein is removed and reversed before reimplantation, thus rendering the venous valves ineffective. There is little to choose between the two methods. More recently very extensive grafting has been performed taking the lower end of the graft down to the tibial or peroneal level and even to the ankle or dorsum of the foot (femorotibial grafts) with a variable success rate. These operations are chiefly for gangrene and any success means avoidance of amputation. Unfortunately some patients have multiple reconstructions which fail and end with amputation which would probably have been best as the first procedure, usually below the knee joint. Unfortunately after most graft failures the patient usually needs an above-knee amputation.

Although the autogenous long saphenous vein is the best graft material for femoropopliteal bypass grafting, in at least a quarter of patients it cannot be used. It may be too small (4–5 mm in diameter seems to be the crucial size), it may be varicose, although a little dilatation is good, it may have been removed in a stripping operation or locally there may be anatomical variations that prevent the full length of the vein being used. Nowadays the veins have sometimes been removed for cardiac grafting in the treatment of heart disease.

Many types of prosthesis have been tried for femoropoplitcal bypass, such as dacron, teflon, bovine arteries and umbilical veins, but none of these has stood the test of time. Graft failure follows occlusion by thrombosis and infection and in the natural grafts aneurysm formation. At present the most favoured plastic prosthesis is made of polytetrafluoroethylene (PTFE, GORETEX) with reinforcing plastic rings that stop occlusion with joint movement. The results of femoropopliteal grafting reported in the literature are very variable. The aim should be to have 90% of patients leaving hospital with patent grafts with a fall off in patency of approximately 10% per annum so that after 5 years it is unlikely that more than 40–50% of grafts are likely to be patent. Plastic grafts fare worse than autogenous grafts.

ANGIOPLASTY

Angioplasty can be by patch or balloon (Figure 4.6), more often nowadays by balloon, to overcome localized narrowings or occlusion of arteries. Patch angioplasty involves the sewing of a patch of plastic or autogenous vein into an artery to prevent narrowing, usually after an endarterectomy, i.e. coring out atheromatous material. It is still uscd in cases of profunda femoris disease and carotid endarterectomies.

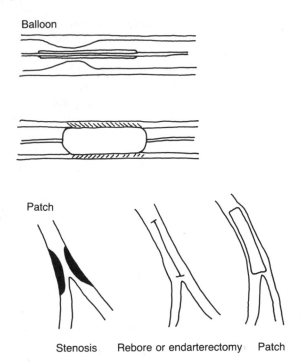

Figure 4.6 Angioplasty.

Balloon angioplasty only became successful after the development of plastic balloons that could be rapidly inflated under considerable pressure but only up to a fixed diameter, usually 6–7mm. The procedure is used for localized stenosis, for example, of a renal artery causing hypertension. It is most successful in large arteries like the aorta and iliac arteries and is now the procedure of choice for limited disease. If it fails or the blockage recurs after a variable interval it can often be performed again. The procedure is relatively non-invasive compared with the surgical operation, may take only half an hour and be performed often as a day case procedure. First a guide wire is inserted into the artery over which the deflated balloon is threaded through the stenosis or localized occlusion (up to 10cm long). The balloon may be passed distally or proximally and in some cases over the aortic bifurcation to reach the contralateral artery. In cases of stenosis of the aortic bifurcation two balloons may be passed via the femoral arteries. Once through the stenosis or occlusion the balloon is inflated suddenly and forcibly with or without the aid of an injection pump. The atheromatous material is forcibly compressed by the balloon and it is unusual for any debris to be liberated as peripheral emboli. Radiographs before and after dilatation reveal the adequacy of the dilatation. If peripheral pulses return the result is likely to be excellent. Assessment of the pressure index before or after dilatation is useful. Following the dilatation the patient is instructed to take 30 mg of aspirin daily and indefinitely in the hope of deterring recurrence from platelet accretion. The larger the vessel and the more localized the stenosis or occlusion the better the result. Dilatation of iliac vessels is likely to be successful in 90% of cases over 3 years. Below the inguinal ligament the results are not as good, 75% of cases over 3 years in some cases of intermittent claudication but less satisfactory results have been found by some investigators (Campbell, 1986; Cole *et al.*, 1987).

Details of arterial reconstructions are given in Greenhalgh (1984).

REFERENCES

Campbell, W.B. (1987) Angioplasty for intermittent claudication. *Br. Med. J.*, **293**, 1047–1048.

Cole, S.E., Baird, R.N., Horrocks, M. and Jeans, W.D. (1987) The role of balloon angioplasty in the management of lower limb ischaemia. *Eur. J. Surg.*, **1**, 61–65.

Greenhalgh, R.M. (Ed.) (1984) *Vascular Surgical Techniques*. Butterworth, London.

Kenney, D.A., Sauvage, L.R. and Wood, S.J. (1983) Comparison of noncrimped externally supported (EXS) and crimped, nonsupported Dacron prostheses for axillofemoral and above knee femoropopliteal bypass. *Surgery*, **92**, 931–946.

Skotnicki, S.H., Buskens, F.G.M. and Reinherts, H.H.M. (eds) (1985) *Recent Advances in Vascular Grafting*. System 4 Associates, Buckinghamshire, UK.

5

Level selection techniques and amputation

The primary objective of limb amputation is to remove sufficient diseased, infected and gangrenous tissue to permit the stump to heal but at the same time retain adequate limb length for prosthetic fitting on suitable patients. A successful amputation is therefore one that is at the lowest possible level and heals primarily. In the late 1940s, 90% of all amputations were at the above-knee level (Murdoch, 1967). Since that time many authors have described the importance of preserving the knee joint and its implications for successful rehabilitation on a prosthesis. Despite these benefits many surgeons associate the below-knee amputation with a high failure rate (Burgess *et al.*, 1982) and are more likely to choose the above-knee level which has a higher healing rate (Barnes *et al.*, 1981).

Recent UK data on amputees referred to a limb centre, show that the above-knee percentage in 1985 was 49% and the below-knee percentage was 42% (Ham *et al.*, 1989). At informed centres the figures reported are very different, for example 31% above knee and 62% below knee (Murdoch *et al.*, 1988). Romano and Burgess (1971) found that most below-knee amputations for vascular disease will heal below the knee and that delayed healing of the stump has not been followed by recurrent ulceration of the stump on weight bearing, suggesting that stump circulation may improve after wound healing and that skin appearance may improve in time and with prosthetic use.

Historically, amputation was thought of as an operation which was dangerous, life saving and had surgical status. Today the emphasis is on arterial reconstruction so amputation is regarded as a failure and is often left to junior staff who are inexperienced and unsupervised. Amputation marks not the end of the story but rather the beginning (Murdoch,

1967) and should be regarded as a part of plastic surgical procedure and therefore a constructive and not a destructive procedure. The difference between healing and non-healing can depend upon the surgical care in handling poorly vascularized tissues (Romano and Burgess, 1971).

When a surgeon has a better knowledge of the total rehabilitation of the patient and the responsibility of the surgeon does not end at the time the sutures are removed, the surgeon's approach becomes more conservative (Romano and Burgess, 1971). The amputating surgeon must realize that the stump has no valid existence on its own and that to become functional a prosthesis is necessary, so contact with a team provides a positive environment of surgery and subsequent successful rehabilitation (Chapter 6). The importance of a settled dedicated team cannot be stressed enough (Cummings et al., 1988).

All patients who are clinically and anatomically acceptable should be considered for arterial reconstruction (Porter et al., 1981) or at least revascularization of the profunda femoris artery as a major collateral source (Moore et al., 1972). Some authors report that previous arterial reconstruction adversely affects the ultimate amputation level (Kazmers et al., 1980) but others report that the benefits of successful revascularization far outweigh the risks of failure and the results are superior to patients undergoing primary amputation (Raviola et al., 1982). For a graft to be cost-effective it must be patent for one year (Gregg, 1985) and the cost of an uncomplicated bypass operation and primary amputation are almost equal when the cost of a prosthesis is included (Raviola et al., 1988). It must, however, be remembered that the criteria for reconstruction and primary amputation vary enormously in both national practices and internationally and data should be interpreted with this in mind.

There is a large potential for limb salvage for the patients with atherosclerosis so the vascular surgeon should be an integral part of the amputee team (Malone et al., 1979). In some hospitals amputations are carried out by orthopaedic surgeons who must be aware of the limb salvage potential and sensitive to its implications in limb surgery (Burgess, 1968). When amputation is the only choice available, surgeons are urged to save the knee joint whenever possible (Burgess and Matsen, 1981; McCollum et al., 1988) and for this to be achieved and the wound to heal, methods of assessment have been developed to add objective information to the surgeon's clinical findings. The assessment techniques include angiography, presence of a popliteal pulse, segmental blood pressure, radioisotope clearance, thermography, transcutaneous oxygen tension and laser Doppler flowmetry. These techniques will now be briefly discussed.

ANGIOGRAPHY

Angiography provides static, anatomical images of the arterial tree from which vessel patency may be determined (Douglas, 1990). No information regarding the dynamics of blood flow is revealed and there are few reported studies relating angiographic findings to amputation level selection. Lim *et al.* (1967) was unable to demonstrate any significant difference between the angiograms of the amputations that healed or failed in their retrospective study. In both groups half the patients had severe or total occlusion of the superficial femoral arteries. Sixty-eight per cent of the successful below-knee group had occluded popliteal arteries compared with 83% of those that failed. Angiography shows no consistent relationship between the severity of the vascular insufficiency and failure of the below-knee amputation to heal and it may also indicate amputation at a higher level when a lower level would have healed (Burgess *et al.*, 1971). If angiography is relied upon to determine amputation levels, the knee joint will be sacrificed needlessly (Romano and Burgess, 1971).

PRESENCE OF THE POPLITEAL PULSE

Many authors agree that the absence of the popliteal pulse is no criterion for level selection as this is evidence of major arterial flow and not the collateral circulation, which is also a major factor in the wound healing of the ischaemic limb (Lim *et al.*, 1967; Barnes *et al.*, 1976). If the presence of the popliteal pulse is relied upon the knee joint will be lost regularly (Romano and Burgess, 1971; Burgess and Matsen, 1981).

SEGMENTAL ARTERIAL BLOOD PRESSURE

Determining systolic blood pressure in the leg using a cuff and Doppler ultrasound transducer is a simple measurement that is performed in many hospitals and consequently it has been extensively investigated as an objective measure of amputation wound healing (Barnes *et al.*, 1976; Pollock and Ernest, 1980). Assumptions have to be made that the major arteries under the cuff are compressible and that arterial systolic pressure is the primary determinant of wound healing (Douglas, 1990).

Pollock and Ernest (1980) recommend pressures greater than 55 mmHg at the incision site and 70 mmHg at the ankle for a below-knee amputation to heal satisfactorily. Other authors suggest different guidelines. Barnes *et al.* (1976) recommended that 70 mmHg was the critical pressure required for a below-knee amputation to heal and Raines *et al.* (1976) recommended a below-knee pressure greater than 65 mmHg combined with an ankle pressure of at least 30 mmHg. Another study failed to demonstrate any correlation between arterial pressure and below-knee healing, reporting that 90% of limbs with no measurable pressure healed (Barnes *et al.*, 1981).

SKIN PERFUSION PRESSURE

The pressure required to stop blood flow in the skin is known as the skin perfusion pressure (SSP). Some authors have found this a useful method to predict healing at below-knee level. Holstein *et al.* (1979) measured the local SPP pre-operatively, i.e. the external pressure required to stop isotope washout using Iodine 133–1 or 125–1 antipyrine mixed with histamine. When the SPP was greater than 30 mmHg, 90% of below-knee amputations healed. If the pressure was less than 20 mmHg only 25% healed. Other authors quote higher readings for success. The method is invasive and although it correlates to a degree with the success of amputation the results are not absolute (Burgess and Matsen, 1981).

RADIOISOTOPE CLEARANCE

Radioisotope clearance has found widespread use in amputation level determination because it allows quantitative skin blood flow to be measured (Douglas, 1990). Authors have used xenon-133 to measure the blood flow and found that there was a sharp end point between success and failure of the stump healing. Readings greater than 2.6 ml/min/100 g tissue lead to primary healing of below-knee amputations (Malone *et al.*, 1981; Moore *et al.*, 1981; Burgess and Matsen, 1981). Later reports suggest that a unique level of skin blood flow for healing does not exist and this is probably due to the fact that xenon has a high affinity for fatty tissue and if clearance is slow, diffusion into the subcutaneous fat increases. Other isotopes have been used (Douglas, 1990).

INFRA-RED THERMOGRAPHY

In a thermogram, the temperature gradients are portrayed pictorially and are directly related to the blood flow in the skin (Douglas, 1990).

Authors recommend gradients of between 2 and 6°C from the proximal to the distal part of the limb (Henderson and Hackett, 1978; Spencer *et al.*, 1981). The method has received little attention and this may be due to the expense of the equipment.

TRANSCUTANEOUS OXYGEN TENSION

Transcutaneous oxygen tension ($TcpO_2$) measured in adult skin is dependent on skin blood flow and therefore this non-invasive technique has attracted interest as a method for predicting amputation healing (Matsen *et al.*, 1980; Burgess *et al.*, 1982; Butler, 1986; Wyss *et al.*, 1988). Reports typically define a critical value below which below-knee amputations are likely to fail. There is some variation in the value and this is thought to be due to the oximeter (Spencer *et al.*, 1985) and the position of the patient during the measurement. Although critical values may vary from 10 to 50 mmHg this is the most widely used objective method of determining amputation healing (Douglas, 1990).

LASER DOPPLER FLOWMETRY

Laser Doppler flowmetry is a technique that gives quantitative measurement of micro-circulatory (capillary) perfusion. Since 1983 it has been applied as a technique to evaluate quantitatively amputation level selection (Holloway and Burgess, 1983; Douglas, 1990). As blood is the bearer of nutrients to and from the skin, capillary perfusion provides the closest assessment of intracellular biochemical activity possible today (Holloway, 1989). It is non-invasive, simple to use and provides a real time measure of perfusion. It compares well with transcutaneous oxygen tension measurements and it may increasingly be used on the feet, accommodating their surface irregularities.

Although there are many factors which influence amputation healing, adequate cutaneous perfusion below the knee remains an essential requirement. Consequently the techniques that measure skin perfusion pressure, oxygen tension and blood flow have proved to be the most valuable indicators of healing (Douglas, 1990). These objective assessment techniques will therefore help in choosing the correct level for amputation but for the stump to heal satisfactorily, the surgery must be good and the post-operative management appropriate and up to date. If the level assessment is in error or the surgery fails, the rehabilitation time is doubled (Murdoch, 1977).

AMPUTATION

The modern amputation is a precision operation aimed at removing diseased or damaged tissue and producing an adequately shaped stump of correct length. It should not be considered as the simple ablation of a limb but rather as an operation designed to construct a new organ of locomotion (Vitali *et al.*, 1967). If performed properly it will result in easy and successful prosthetic fitting and will provide balanced, effective muscular power for locomotion and propulsion of the prosthesis.

Care in the operative technique is essential and healing can depend upon the careful handling of these poorly vascularized and nourished tissues. The management of the skin which should ideally have normal sensation, is the basis of success and it should always be handled gently and closed with close abutment and sutured without tension. Vigorous skin retraction and the use of forceps must be avoided. Myoplastic techniques should be used where the skin flaps include muscle, so that the blood supply between skin and muscle flaps is not severed and there is the advantage of producing a physiologically stable stump in which the vascular dynamics are efficient. This type of stump is firm, cylindrical, more powerful, capable of proprioceptive sensation with less likelihood of muscle wasting and a prominent bone end and able to be comfortably fitted into modern prostheses.

The cut bone end should be sculptured and smoothed before closure and all debris washed away. The nerves should be cut high under tension to avoid a neuroma forming at the site of the scar. The major blood vessels should be ligated individually and low to ensure survival of the maximum number of collaterals and haemostasis. Suction drains should be used for approximately 48 hours when drainage is generally complete. A period of use longer than this can lead to infection. Tourniquets are generally only necessary with the non-vascular patients. (The preparations for surgery are discussed in Chapter 7.)

Digital and partial foot

Digital and forefoot amputations are indicated where the blood supply to the foot is adequate, as shown by palpable pedal pulses, Doppler insonation and angiography. It may be necessary after a successful arterial reconstruction or lumbar sympathectomy and after trauma where a digit or part of the forefoot is dead, although, surprisingly, some tissues apparently near death are revascularized successfully. In diabetics limited amputation of digits or the forefoot may often be

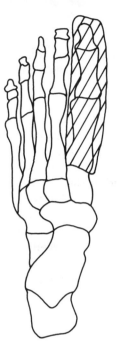

Figure 5.1 Ray amputation.

successful in gaining healing. Where the major components in gangrene are infection and neuropathy, atherosclerosis plays a lesser part. The greater the atherosclerotic element, the less likely healing is to be achieved. Any or all the digits may be amputated and, if necessary with removal of one or more metatarsals, especially if they or their joints are involved by infection, osteomyelitis or pyarthrosis. If the phalanges and metatarsals are removed, this is called a 'ray amputation' (Figure 5.1).

The principle in such limited amputations is to cut directly down to bone proximal to necrotic tissues without any formal flap dissection. The bones and any necrotic tissues are literally 'filleted out' rather than dissected. Abscesses are drained and dead tissue, such as tendons and fascia, are removed. Usually the wound edges are only lightly approximated or left to heal by granulation.

Partial foot amputations such as the Lisfranc, a tarsometatarsal disarticulation (Figure 5.2) and Chopart, a mid-tarsal amputation (Figure 5.3) are only of historical interest, or very rarely may be practised after trauma where the blood supply proximally is normal. Prosthetic fitting is difficult for such amputations as the muscular

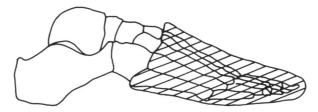

Figure 5.2 Lisfranc amputation.

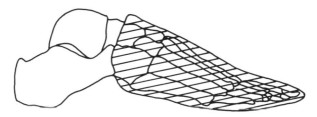

Figure 5.3 Chopart amputation.

imbalance may lead to an equinus deformity of the foot due to the strength of the tendo calcaneum and lack of distal attachment of the dorsiflexors. Traditionally both are fitted with a leather bootee which fits into a normal shoe. In some cases surgical shoes with appropriate inserts and rocker soles are fitted.

Syme

The Syme amputation, as originally described in 1842, is a disarticulation through the ankle joint by two incisions, anterior and plantar (Figure 5.4). The anterior incision is through the ankle joint to allow for disarticulation of the talus and section of the lower end of the tibia and fibula and the plantar incision is around the calcaneum. The talus and calcaneum are then dissected out and the skin flap from the heel is used to cover the bone ends. Often the amputation is performed in two stages and the scar is anterior. There have been numerous modifications to the original description but the amputation has had little success in the management of the vascular patient with vascular disease. Its use in traumatic cases, frost bite, leprosy and chronic infection has been more successful. Patients generally start to bear weight 4 weeks post-operatively unless the wound is enclosed in plaster of Paris, when this

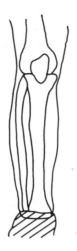

Figure 5.4 Syme amputation.

may be earlier. The resultant stump is weight bearing and amputees are able to walk short distances in their own home without a prosthesis and with a slight limp. Less energy is required to walk, and as the epiphyseal plate is retained, it is suitable for growing children. The conventional leather prosthesis is bulky, adds width to the malleoli and is therefore cosmetically poor, especially for a young woman. The modern close-fitting Syme prosthesis, which is not totally end bearing, is more cosmetically acceptable.

Two similar operations of historical interest are those of Pirogoff and Boyd. With the Pirogoff amputation (Figure 5.5) the posterior third of the calcaneum is arthodesed to the tibia which produces a longer stump than the Syme and therefore less of a limp. With the Boyd amputation (Figure 5.6), the incision is made below the lateral malleolus and base

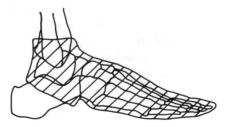

Figure 5.5 Pirogoff amputation.

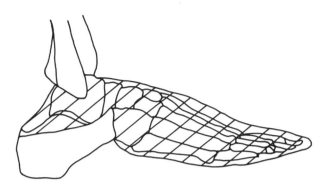

Figure 5.6 Boyd amputation.

of the metatarsals. Articular cartilage is removed and the calcaneum brought forward until the weight-bearing surface of the heel is under the long axis of the leg. Steinman pins or Kirschner wires are used to provide internal fixation. The prosthesis is the same as for the Syme but the leg is slightly longer. The procedure is popular in Scandinavia. Shoe fitting is a major problem with these two amputation levels.

Transtibial or below knee

The most dramatic change in modern times has been the greater drive to amputate below the knee started by Kendrick (1954), who showed the effectiveness of the long posterior flap in below-knee amputation, later popularized by Burgess (1971) and modified by the use of the sagittal method (Persson, 1974). Below-knee amputation using equal flaps has a bad reputation because of failure of wound healing, usually due to necrosis of the anterior flap. Using the long posterior flap method this was to an extent overcome but the stump was often deformed by large 'dog ears' and although it looks satisfactory in the recumbent situation when the leg was flexed at the knee joint, the soft tissues fall back and leave the tibial bony crest exposed under the skin. Pressure there quite often led to ulceration and the need to reshape the stump. The subcutaneous bony end was often extremely tender and made for difficulty in prosthetic fitting. The modern 'skew flap' method (McCollum *et al.*, 1985) ensures that the scar of the amputation is obliquely situated in such a way that the blood supply to the flaps is at its maximum (Robinson *et al.*, 1982). The covering of the lower end of the tibia by the pared down soleus and gastrocnemius muscles covers and

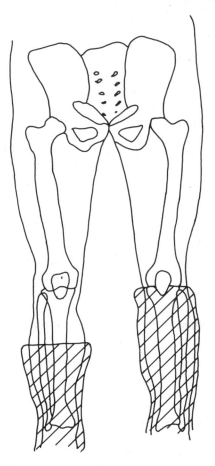

Figure 5.7 Transtibial amputation (left) and knee disarticulation (right).

protects the underlying tibial crest from pressure from the prosthesis. The hemispherical end from the conclusion of the operation permits early casting to take place.

The ideal length of a below-knee stump for modern prosthetics is 14 cm from the tibial plateau (Figure 5.7). Stumps that are less than 8 cm are difficult to fit with a below-knee prosthesis. Some surgeons divide the lower leg into three, two-thirds are removed and one-third remains. This ensures that tall patients are left with stumps that are in proportion with their size. Other surgeons amputate at the largest part of the calf muscle for exactly the same reason. Patients with knee flexion contractures greater than 15 degrees may be unable to be fitted satisfactorily with an effective below-knee walking prosthesis. Patients who have a fixed knee flexion contracture of more than 30 degrees are generally regarded as being unsuitable for a below-knee amputation. Also, patients who are unable to make use of the knee joint functionally because of senility, perhaps a CVA with resultant spasticity or because they are have no rehabilitation potential are also unsuitable for a BK. The importance of the patient's vascular state has been described earlier.

In the past the prosthesis consisted of a leather thigh corset and side steel supports and a metal or wooden leg piece. These are still used for patients with short or scarred stumps and those unable to bear weight on the patella tendon. The more common prosthesis for this level today is the patella tendon bearing (PTB) prosthesis which has been used since 1959. Patients are able to take a substantial amount of their total weight on the patella tendon area. Accurate socket fitting and alignment are essential with this prosthesis (see Chapter 12).

Stump shrinkage generally takes place for 6–12 months following amputation but it may continue for up to 2 years. With the PTB prosthesis adjustments have to be made during this period to accommodate the changing volume of the stump. Function is usually excellent and patients with bilateral below-knee amputations are often able to walk with or without the help of sticks.

Knee disarticulation or through knee

Operation at this level is quick and relatively bloodless and is generally used for the severely ill patient with peripheral vascular disease or for those who will never walk. No bone is cut and wound healing is not a problem if equal lateral flaps are used (Figure 5.7). In the past a long anterior flap was used which led to tissue necrosis. The skin flaps, however, have to be almost as long as for the below-knee amputation. The patella is preserved and the menisci generally removed and the patella tendon is sutured to the cruciate ligaments or posterior capsule. The scar should avoid the weight-bearing area and tight skin closure should be avoided and drains used. For the chairbound amputee the extra length of the intact femur helps with balance and functional activities. For the active amputee the long lever provides extra strength and the large weight-bearing surface provides excellent proprioceptive sensation. In the young, preservation of the distal femoral epiphysis allows the femur to grow normally. As there is little muscle atrophy with this amputation early fitting is possible. The prosthesis is less cosmetic than that supplied for an above-knee amputee because the bulbous femoral condyles have to be accommodated and the articulated knee protrudes beyond the natural knee when sitting. However, development of the four bar linkage knee joint and swing phase control has helped.

Gritti-Stokes

The femur is transected above the condyles and the patella, denuded of cartilage, is attached to the end of the femur with the aim that end weight bearing should be possible. It takes time for the 'fracture' to unite and weight bearing is seldom achieved as often there is non-union

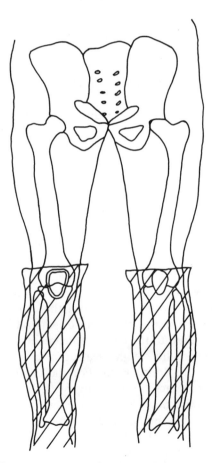

Figure 5.8 Gritti–Stoke amputation (left) and Slocum amputation (right).

of the patella which often retracts upwards due to the pull of the quadriceps. The amputation technique uses a long posterior flap and skin closure is easier than with knee disarticulation as the stump end is not bulbous. However, the femoral epiphysis is lost and the length of the limb means there is also insufficient space to locate a knee control device at this level and its use is not recommended by prosthetists. A similar operation was described by Callender-Long in 1933 and Slocum in 1949 which removed the femoral condyles and the patella. The prosthetic disadvantages of the operation are as for the Gritti-Stokes (Figure 5.8).

Transfemoral or above knee

An above-knee stump must allow 13 cm above the opposite knee line for a prosthetic knee articulation, but otherwise be as long as possible, the ideal being 25–30 cm from the greater trochanter (Figure 5.9). If the thigh length is divided into three, it is recommended that one-third is removed. As with the below-knee amputation this ensures that the height of the patient is taken into consideration. For successful prosthetic fitting, hip flexion deformities should be no more than 10 degrees but a maximum of 30 degrees may be accommodated. The flaps should be anterior/posterior and equal in length. Adequate skin should be available to ensure suturing can take place without tension. The cut bone end should be sculptured and smoothed before the muscle is sutured. Arteries and veins should be ligated separately to ensure that maximum numbers of collateral vessels survive. Closed suction drains are used. A myoplastic stump is very important as it is prosthetically more satisfactory, more powerful, the bone end is well buried and there is a better stump to socket relationship. The healing rate of the above-knee amputation is good and as there is much soft tissue, the stump is easy to fit within a socket. The above-knee stump has a tendency to abduct, especially with a more proximal amputation. A full exercise programme should ensure that a contracture does not develop. The rehabilitation time is less than that of the below-knee amputation but the energy required for walking is much greater. The distal epiphysis has been removed and the stump is not end bearing. For the older patient the prosthesis is weight bearing at the ischial tuberosity with a pelvic band and shoulder strap and the socket is built to take the shape of the thigh. For the younger patient the prosthesis may have a suction socket and be self-suspending with no pelvic band being necessary. For the fitter patient a variety of knee devices are available for walking with a free knee and taking weight on a flexed knee (see Chapter 12).

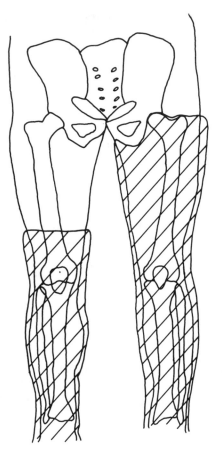

Figure 5.9 Transfemoral amputation and hip disarticulation.

Hip disarticulation and hindquarter

These amputations are generally performed for malignancy, but some are necessary for trauma and failed hip surgery and ischaemic above-knee amputation stumps. With the hip disarticulation the scar is located anteriorly to avoid faecal contamination. The tissue should be handled very gently and shock is likely due to the volume of blood loss. Muscles are cut at their origins rather than in their vascular parts. Complications of the operation include haemorrhage and haematoma. For the hemipelvectomy or hindquarter, the operation is performed in side lying position and the bone is divided at the sacroiliac joint and half an inch lateral to the pubic symphysis. A long posterior flap is used and the prosthesis is either the tilting table or Canadian tilting table. Both require extensive pelvic suspension and these patients are encouraged to use crutches as soon as possible after the operation. Sitting is easier after the hip articulation as the ischial tuberosity is preserved (Figure 5.9).

POST-OPERATIVE MANAGEMENT

Adequate analgesia must be ~~to be~~ prescribed for the immediate post-operative period. For reasons ~~already~~ stated in Chapter 7, it should be administered routinely to prevent pain rather than treat it once it has arisen. Concurrent diseases will continue to be treated and the course of antibiotics continued. Management in the post-operative period is described in Chapter 7 and rehabilitation in Chapter 8.

REFERENCES

Barnes, R.W., Shanik, G.D. and Slaymaher, E.E. (1976) An index of healing in below-knee amputations: leg blood pressure by Doppler Ultrasound. *Surgery*, **79**, 13–20.

Barnes, R.W., Thornhill, B., Nix, L., Rittgers, E. and Turley, G. (1981) Prediction of amputation wound healing. *Arch. Surg.*, **116**, 80–83.

Burgess, E.M. (1968) Stabilisation of muscles in lower extremity amputations. *J. Bone Joint Surg.*, **50A**, 1486–1487.

Burgess, E.M. and Matsen, F.A. (1981) Determining amputation levels in Peripheral Vascular Disease. *J. Bone Joint Surg.*, **63A**, 1493–1497.

Burgess, E.M., Romano, R.L., Zettl, J.H. and Schrock, R.D. (1971) Amputation of the leg for peripheral vascular insufficiency. *J. Bone Joint Surg.*, **531**, 874–890.

Burgess, E.M., Matsen, F.A., Wyss, C.R. and Simmons, C.W. (1982) Segmental transcutaneous measurements of pO_2 in patients requiring below-knee amputations for peripheral insufficiency. *J. Bone Joint Surg.*, **70A**, 203–207.

Butler, C.M. (1986) The vascular amputee. MS Thesis, University of London.

Cummings, J.G.R., Spence, V.A., Jain, A.S., McCollum, P.T., Stewart, C., Walker, W.F. and Murdoch, G. (1988) Further experience in the healing rate of lower limb amputations. *Eur. J. Vasc. Surg.*, **2**, 383–385.

Douglas, S.L.E. (1990) Laser Doppler flowmetry. *In-vitro* quantification and use in amputation surgery. PhD Thesis, University of London.

Gregg, R.O. (1985) Bypass or amputation? Concomitant review of bypass arterial grafting and major amputation. *Am. J. Surg.*, **149**, 397–402.

Ham, R.O., Luff, R. and Roberts, V.C. (1989) A five year review of referrals for prosthetic treatment in England, Wales and Northern Ireland 1981–1985. *Health Trends*, **21**, 3–6.

Henderson, H.P. and Hackett, M.E.J.V. (1978) Value of thermography in pvd. *Angio*, **29**, 65–75.

Holloway, G.A. (1989) Amputation level selection by laser Doppler flowmetry, in *Lower Extremity Amputation* (eds W.S. Moore and J.M. Malone), Saunders, London.

Holloway, G.A. and Burgess, E.M. (1983) Preliminary experiences with laser Doppler velocimetry for the determination of amputation levels. *Prosthet. Orthot. Int.*, **7**, 63–66.

Holstein, P., Dovey, H. and Lassen, N.A. (1979) Wound healing in above knee amputation in relation to skin perfusion pressure. *Acta Orthop. Scand.*, **50**, 59–66.

Kazmers, M., Satiani, B. and Evans, W.E. (1987) Amputation level following unsuccessful distal limb salvage operations. *Surgery*, **87**, 683–687.

Kendrick, R.R. (1954) Below-knee amputation in arteriosclerotic gangrene. *Br. J. Surg.*, **44**, 13–17.

Lim, R.C., Blaisdell, F.W., Hall, A., Moore, A.D. and Thomas, W.S. (1967) Below knee amputation for ischaemic gangrene. *Surg. Gynae. Obst.*, **125**, 493–501.

McCollum, P.T., Spence, V.A., Walker, W.F. and Murdoch, G. (1985) A rationale for skew flaps in below-knee amputation surgery. *Prosthet. Orthot. Int.*, **9**, 95–99.

McCollum, P.T., Spence, V.A. and Walker, W.F. (1988) Amputation for PVD: the case for level selection *Br. J. Surg.*, **75**, 1193–1195.

Malone, J.M., Moore, W.S., Goldstone, J. and Malone, S.J. (1979) Therapeutic and economic impact of a modern amputation programme. *Ann. Surg.*, **189**, 798–802.

Malone, J.M., Moore, W., Leal, J.M. and Childers, S.J. (1981) Rehabilitation for lower extremity amputation. *Arch. Surg.*, **116**, 93–98.

Matsen, F.A., Wyss, C.R., Pedegana, L.R. *et al.* (1980) Transcutaneous oxygen tension measurement in Peripheral Vascular Disease. *Surg. Gynae. Obst.*, **150**, 525–528.

Moore, W.S., Hall, A.D. and Lim, R.C. (1972) Below knee amputation for ischaemic gangrene. *Am. J. Surg.*, **124**, 123–134.

Moore, W.S., Henry, R.E., Malone, J.M. *et al.* (1981) Prospective use of Xenon Xe-133 clearance for amputation level selection. *Arch. Surg.*, **116**, 86–88.

Murdoch, G. (1967) Levels of amputation and limiting factors. *Ann. R. Coll. Surg.*, **40**, 204–216.

Murdoch, G. (1977) Amputation surgery in the lower extremity. *Prosthet. Orthot. Int.*, **1**, 72–83.

Murdoch, G., Condie, D.N., Gardner D., Ramsay, E., Smith, A., Stewart, C.P.U., Swanson, A.J.G. and Troup, I.M. (1988) The Dundee experience, in *Amputation Surgery and Lower Limb Prosthetics*, Blackwell Scientific, Oxford., pp. 440–457.

Persson, B.M. (1974) Sagittal incision for below-knee amputation in ischaemic gangrene. *J. Bone Joint Surg.*, **56B**, 110–114.

Pollock, S.B. and Ernest, C.B. (1980) Use of Doppler pressure measurements in predicting success in amputation of the leg. *Am. J. Surg.*, **139**, 303–306.

Porter, J.M., Baur, G.M. and Taylor, L.M. (1981) Lower extremity amputation for ischaemia. *Arch. Surg.*, **116**, 89–92.

Raines, R.W., Darling, R.C. and Ruth, J. (1976) Vascular laboratory criteria for the management of peripheral vascular disease of the lower extremities. *Surgery*, **79**, 21–28.

Raviola, C.A., Nichter, L., Baker, J.D., Busittil, R.W., Barker, W.F., Machleder, H.I. and Moore, W.S. (1982) Femoropopliteal tibial bypass; What price failure? *Am. J. Surg.*, **144**, 115–123.

Raviola, C.A., Nichter, L.S., Baker, J.D., Busuttil, R.W., Machleder, H.I. and Moore, W.S. (1988) Cost of treating advanced leg aschaemia. Bypass grafts *vs* primary amputation. *Arch. Surg.*, **123**, 495–496.

Robinson, K.P., Hoile, R. and Coddington, T. (1982) Skew flap myoplastic below knee amputation: A preliminary report. *Br. J. Surg.*, **69**, 554–557.

Romano, R.L. and Burgess, E.M. (1971) Level selection in lower extremity amputation. *Clin. Orth.*, **74**, 177–184.

Spencer, V.A., Walker, W.F., Troup, I.M. and Murdoch, G. (1981) Amputation of the ischaemic limb: selection of the optimum site by thermography. *Angio*, **32**, 155–169.

Spencer, V.A., McCollum, P.T., McGregor, I.W., Sherwin, S.J. and Walker, W.F. (1985) The effects of the transcutaneous electrode on the variability of dermal oxygen change. *Clin. Phys. Physiol. Meas.*, **6**, 139–145.

Vitali, M., Harris, E.E. and Redhead, R.G. (1967) Amputees and their prostheses in action. *Ann. Rev. Con. Surg. (Eng.)*, **40**, 260–266.

Wyss, C.R., Harrington, R.M., Burgess, E.M. and Matsen, F.A. (1988) Transcutaneous oxygen tension as a predictor of success after an amputation. *J. Bone Joint Surg.*, **70A**, 203–207.

6

The team approach

THE MULTIDISCIPLINARY CLINICAL TEAM

Introduction

Multidisciplinary clinical teams (MDCT) have developed gradually over many years. The earliest were found in psychiatric hospitals and in those caring for the mentally handicapped, but early examples can also be seen in the acute hospitals, where, for example, in the operating theatres such team work is essential. The need for the MDCT has developed as medicine and rehabilitation have both developed. Advances in science have widened the knowledge of aetiology and methods of investigation and treatment. New disciplines of staff have subsequently arisen in the light of these advances and their place and contribution is now unquestioned. Increasingly research, diagnosis, care and also treatment have become multidisciplinary (Batchelor and McFarlane, 1980a, b).

A team can be defined as a group of two or more health professionals from different disciplines who share common values and work towards common objectives (Halstead, 1976). The major objective of the MDCT is therefore to co-ordinate plans of care that have been evolved by different health workers; an effective team functions as a team and not as a group of different health professionals (Sanders, 1986). Communication and flexible personalities are vital for good results as each team member is dependent on the other; no one person can meet all the patient's needs. For good team interaction it is essential that each team member earns the trust and confidence of the others by consistently demonstrating competence in their individual area of expertise (Mensch and Ellis, 1987). This makes the necessary overlapping of work possible and the resentment felt by the invasion of another individual's work avoidable (Jamieson and Hill, 1976).

The following points are essential for good multidisciplinary clinical team work:

1. personal relationships;
2. good professional co-operation and flexibility;
3. agreed team objectives;
4. allocation by each member of a sufficient amount of time to pursue the objectives;
5. regular meetings that are well attended;
6. no professional should be held responsible for the negligence of another;
7. high standards of patient confidentiality within the team members;
8. co-ordination by communication, planning and monitoring;
9. team members should have the experience and status to match the demands of the particular team in the interest of preserving the balance and there should be mutual respect for each other's skills and opinions;
10. there is a likelihood of roles overlapping but it is important to distinguish each team member's role;
11. unit policies such as ward round, patient routines, discharge, etc. should be discussed regularly; and
12. adequate administrative or clerical co-ordination and a defined geographical base should be available (Batchelor and McFarlane, 1980a; Furnell *et al.*, 1987).

Membership, co-ordination and leadership

The MDCT may have a different membership for each clinical case although there will always be a stable core of professionals working together. Each member makes a different contribution with different patients, depending upon the individual patient's needs. The MDCT may be large and it is therefore essential for there to be a focal point or a co-ordinator. The co-ordinator must be a professional who deals with all or the majority of patients in a specific team and may be the doctor, nurse, therapist or social worker.

In the west, the majority of junior staff are in positions of training and therefore few team members remain in their jobs indefinitely. This, however, is not the case with the chief or consultant surgeon or physician. Following appointment this person will remain in the post for many years and is therefore the only 'team' member who provides genuine continuity of care and directs the unit policy. Doctors should therefore provide unit and policy leadership, but the daily MDCT co-ordination lies in the hands of the professional who deals most closely with that particular case or group of individuals.

This 'leader' should therefore:

1. bring all relevant resources to bear quickly on the individual patient's problem;
2. have the authority to get things done;
3. make the final decision if there is a doubt or disagreement; and
4. carry the overall responsibility, not for other individuals' work but for clinical investigation and treatment of the patient (Batchelor and McFarlane, 1980a, b).

THE AMPUTEE MULTIDISCIPLINARY CLINICAL TEAM

Membership

A team approach to the management of the amputee began during the Second World War in the USA. The influx of amputees led to amputee centres being set up in military general hospitals, providing improved and co-ordinated care for this group of patients. Following the war, the US Veterans Administration extended the team approach into all its hospitals and clinics (Burgess and Alexander, 1973).

In the UK following the Second World War the provision of artificial limbs to both war pensioners and civilian amputees became the responsibility of the Ministry of Health. Artificial Limb and Appliance Centres (ALAC) were opened throughout the country to provide prosthetic care on an out-patient basis. However, it was not until 1965 that a 17 bed in-patient facility adjoining prosthetic out-patient care was opened. This was at Dundee, Scotland, and it was at the time the only centre in Western Europe offering in-patient care exclusively for amputees (Murdoch et al., 1988). Today hospitals are working more closely with the prosthetic centres in their locality.

The amputee team is a multidisciplinary team that treats the medical, physical, psychological, social and vocational aspects of amputation (Goldberg, 1984). The team must work together to motivate the patient to cope with the necessarily tough rehabilitation programme (Chadwick, 1986). Six professionals generally act as the core to the team: the surgeon,

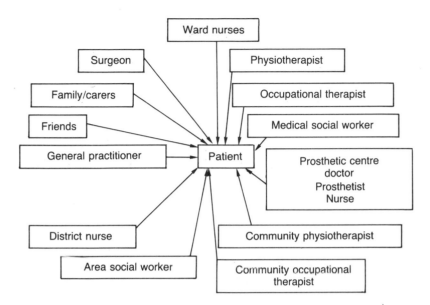

Figure 6.1 The Amputee Team.

physiotherapist, prosthetist, nurse, occupational therapist and social worker. Burgess stressed that the first three members remain the tripod upon which rehabilitation of the lower limb amputee has rested (Burgess and Alexander, 1973). Other members of the team may include a clinical psychologist, a vocational counsellor, a rehabilitation specialist, a disablement resettlement officer and a bioengineer. The major roles and function of each professional will be described (Figure 6.1).

The **surgeon's** role is most important and is to provide a well-healed stump at the lowest possible level, that will enable successful rehabilitation to take place. The surgeon should be trained and experienced in amputation surgery and, as the majority of amputations today are for vascular disease (88%), would generally be a vascular surgeon. The surgeon should have a knowledge of the rehabilitation process and current prostheses, which should ensure that a positive attitude regarding amputation is instilled in the patient and their relatives and that the feeling of failure and defeat is not conveyed. In some cases the surgeon acts as the team co-ordinator and should always stimulate unit policy.

The **physiotherapist** often knows the patient better than any other team member due to involvement in all aspects of the rehabilitation programme from the pre-operative stage to discharge into the community. Daily contact with the patient enables the physiotherapist to become aware of the patient's motivation and concerns, psychologically, socially and physically. The role of the physiotherapist is to mobilize and strengthen the patient and to work with other members of the team to prevent flexion contractures. The physiotherapist uses techniques to retrain the patient's gait which may include the use of immediate post-operative prosthetic fittings or early walking aids and temporary and definitive prostheses. Whether using a prosthesis or a wheelchair, the physiotherapist works with the patient until their final return to the community. The physiotherapist ensures the rehabilitation programme is constantly reviewed and short- and long-term goals are set. This is especially important if the patient remains in an acute hospital bed. Often the physiotherapist acts as co-ordinator to the amputee team and should keep abreast with new developments.

The **prosthetist** may either be employed by the hospital or by a private manufacturing company. The patient and prosthetist often meet early in the pre- or post-operative period and the prosthetist recommends the type of prosthesis with adaptations that are suitable for each individual patient. The prosthetist will measure or cast the stump and fabricate or assist in the fabrication of the prosthesis. Other team members are informed of prosthetic technological developments and new products by the prosthetist. To ensure that the prosthetic fit and alignment are correct, the prosthetist works closely with the physiotherapist.

The major role of the **nurse** is in the pre- and post-operative phases which if managed well, can speed up the patient's rehabilitation progress. The nurse provides support and explanations to the patient and their family in the pre-operative phase. Drugs for pain, infection and diabetes are administered by the nurse, who also controls fluid balance and prepares the patient for the operating theatre. The appropriate dressing care and wound management are applied by the nurse, who also ensures the patient takes a good diet. The nurse continues to practise with the patient the activities learnt during therapy and maintains contact with the family and carers as they visit the ward. As nurses are around the patient for 24 hours every day, good rapport and psychological support are also gained by the patient and relatives from this professional group.

The **occupational therapist's** role is in training or helping the patient regain the everyday activities of daily living. The occupational therapist may loan or order a wheelchair for the patient to use in the pre- and post-prosthetic phase and teach them how to use it functionally. The occupational therapist visits the patient's home and arranges the supply of equipment and technical aids that may be necessary. The patient is ensured the necessary community services required on discharge by the occupational therapist, who also plays a large part in the psychological aspects of amputation and assists the patient and their family to adapt to the amputation, disability and handicap. In the case of the upper limb amputee, the occupational therapist is involved in the functional training of these patients.

The **social worker's** role is initially to provide some emotional and psychological support to the patient and their family and also to give social and financial help when it is necessary. With the increase in numbers of elderly amputees, the social worker's role is expanding. If there are problems with rehousing or if a transfer to long-term care is necessary, the social worker will assist both the patient and their relatives in these cases. The social worker also links up with the community services when discharge is imminent. The psychological information gained by the social worker is vital in influencing the rehabilitation goals and programme (Varghese and Redford, 1982).

In the UK a Disablement Service or Prosthetic Centre medical officer or rehabilitation specialist prescribes the prostheses. In other countries this is done by the prosthetist, the patient having been assessed as a suitable prosthetic wearer by the operating surgeon. The clinical psychologist is involved when an amputee is not showing the normal recovery pattern from the loss of a leg. Counselling may be necessary if the amputee is finding it difficult to come to terms with the loss. The disablement resettlement officer or vocational counsellor helps the patient in their return to work by providing a hospital or vocational link if it is necessary. Financial, physical or social support may also be required. A bioengineer may be involved in the team when new equipment or prosthetic are required. The role of the bioengineer will vary with the nature of work at the centre. The pain control teams in the UK are staffed by doctors (usually anaesthetists) and nurses. Their role is to control and manage the patient's pain in the pre-operative, operative and post-operative phases. The physicist or measurements technician assists the surgeon in the selection of operation level by using a variety of equipment to assess the viability of the limb.

A well-organized and functioning team inspires security and confidence on the part of the patient as well as the group. The composite views and opinions of the team produce higher professional standards and avoid duplication of effort, misunderstanding and time loss (Russek, 1961).

Co-ordination and leadership

As the numbers involved in the amputee team are large it is essential that the good team methods presented earlier prevail. This will ensure the good results and the maximum benefit to the patient that so many authors have described is achieved (Murdoch, 1977; Ham *et al.*, 1987; Dormandy and Thomas, 1988). The large number of team members also makes it easy for no one to take ultimate responsibility for reaching the team objective goals (Jamieson and Hill, 1976). For this and reasons previously described, there should be a team co-ordinator and team leader. Many feel that the leader should be the surgeon and that the surgeon should probably be the co-ordinator, but only if trained to the duties of the other members so that their difficulties are understood and useful advice can be given. This is a task that will daunt any busy surgeon and one which may require considerable tact and diplomacy (Jamieson and Hill, 1976; Hutton and Rothnie, 1977; Varghese and Redford, 1982). In other teams the rehabilitation medicine specialist acts as team leader and sets unit policy. Team or unit plans and policy have to be long term for changes and results to materialize and for this, leadership is necessary. The longest serving team member should act as unit leader and this is generally the chief or consultant surgeon.

Many authors feel that the physical therapist emerges as the key person to co-ordinate on the amputee team (Burgess and Alexander, 1973; Ham *et al.*, 1987). In other centres the occupational therapist acts as co-ordinator and in others the social worker. Local variations will be seen as personalities and the environment and service needs vary.

A review in 1976 reported that team care had become a catch phrase and that there had been very few studies evaluating its benefit (Halstead, 1976). The roles of the three key team members (Burgess and Alexander, 1973), the surgeon, physiotherapist and prosthetist, have been evaluated (Ham *et al.*, 1987). The study found that these members helped to reduce the numbers of above-knee amputations, reduce the hospital in-patient stay, increase the number of patients receiving and being discharged fully rehabilitated on a prosthesis, reduce the need for return physiotherapy visits and increased the functional use of the prosthesis (Ham *et al.*, 1985). The team approach maximized the patients' potential, saved the health district approximately £3500 per patient on bed stay, out-patient physiotherapy and transportation and also increased staff morale as the patients were 'kept moving'.

Summary

The advantages of the team approach are therefore that:

1. all the disciplines work together to maximize the patient's potential;
2. a good prosthetic fitting leading on to full prosthetic training ensures that no artificial legs remain in the cupboard;
3. financial, social, psychological problems are discussed and managed appropriately;
4. the training and education are more attractive and easier to organize; and
5. clinical research is possible and promoted by the positive atmosphere (Varghese and Redford, 1982).

Amputee teams must have a co-ordinator to organize day-to-day plans and a leader to provide unit policy and continuity.

REFERENCES

Batchelor, I. and McFarlane, J. (1980a) *Multidisciplinary Clinical Teams*, Kings Fund Project Paper RC12, pp. 7–21.

Batchelor, I. and McFarlane, J. (1980b) The Multidisciplinary Clinical Team – A Working Paper, pp. 23–34.

Burgess, E.M. and Alexander, A.G. (1973) The expanding role of the physical therapist on the amputee rehabilitation team. *Phys. Ther.*, **53**, 141–143.

Chadwick, S.J.D. (1986) Restoring dignity and mobility in the amputee. *Geriatric Medicine*, July, 43–46.

Dormandy, J.A. and Thomas, P.R.S. (1988) What is the natural history of a critically ischaemic patient with and without his leg?, in *Limb Salvage and Amputation for Vascular Disease* (eds R.M. Greenhalgh, C.W. Jamieson and A.N. Nicolaides), Saunders, London, pp. 11–26.

Furnell J., Flett, S. and Clarke, D.F. (1987) Multidisciplinary Clinical Team: some issues in establishment and function. *Hospital and Health Services Review*, January, 15–18.

Goldberg, R.T. (1984) New trends in the rehabilitation of lower extremity amputees. *Rehabilitation Literature*, **45**, 2–11.

Halstead, L.S. (1976) Team care in chronic illness. A critical review of the literature of the last 25 years. *Arch. Phys. Med. Rehabil.*, **57**, 507–511.

Ham, R.O., Thornberry, D.J., Regan, J.F., Butler, C.M., Davis, B., Cotton, L.T. and Roberts, V.C. (1985) Rehabilitation of the vascular amputee – one method evaluated. *Physiotherapy Practice*, **1**, 6–13.

Ham, R., Regan, J.M. and Roberts, V.C. (1987) Evaluation of introducing the Team Approach to the care of the amputee: the Dulwich Study. *Prosthet. Orthot. Int.*, **11**, 25–30.

Hutton, I.M. and Rothnie, N.G. (1977) The early mobilisation of the elderly amputee. *Br. J. Surg.*, **64**, 267–270.

Jamieson, C.W. and Hill, D. (1976) Amputation for vascular disease. *Br. J. Surg.*, **63**, 683–690.

Mensch, G. and Ellis, P.M. (1987) Preoperative and postoperative care and the responsibilities of the physical therapist, in *Physical Therapy Management of Lower Extremity Amputations,* Heinemann Medical Books, London, pp. 45–96.

Murdoch, G. (1977) Amputation surgery in the lower extremity – part II. *Prosthet. Orthot. Int.*, **1**, 183–192.

Murdoch, G., Condie, D.W., Gardiner, D., Ramsay, E., Smith, A., Stewart, C.P.U., Swanson, A.J.G. and Troup, I.M. (1988) The Dundee experience, in *Amputation Surgery and Lower Limb Prosthetics* (ed. G. Murdoch), Blackwell Scientific, Oxford, pp. 450–457.

Russek, A.S. (1961) Management of lower extremity amputees. *Arch. Phys. Med. Rehabil.*, Oct., 687–705.

Sanders, G.T. (1986) Postoperative management, in *Lower Limb Amputations: a Guide to Rehabilitation*, F.A. Davis, Philadelphia, pp. 357–383.

Varghese, G. and Redford, J.B. (1982) Preoperative assessment and management of amputees, in *Rehabilitation Management of Amputees* (ed. S.N. Banerjee), Rehabilitation Medicine Library, Baltimore, pp. 11–16.

7

Ward management

Ward management of the amputee can be divided into three phases: the pre-amputation phase, the operative phase and the post-amputation phase. It is in these three phases that the nurse has much to contribute to the care and treatment of the amputee patient, ensuring successful return to the community.

PRE-AMPUTATION PHASE

In this initial phase of ward management the prospective amputee may already be in the surgical ward following investigation or treatment for arterial disease, but may, however, have been on a medical or geriatric ward following treatment for diabetes or another manifestation of atherosclerosis, a cerebrovascular accident or heart attack. Whichever is the case, investigations and assessments will be carried out before the operation, all of which will help the nurse plan care for the patient.

The majority of amputations in the western world are for vascular disease and patients presenting with this condition will generally have some insight into the nature of their progressive illness and will have experienced vascular pain. In some cases of vascular disease, for example embolism, the onset will be sudden. For the patients undergoing amputation for a malignancy or congenital deformity the operation will again be a planned 'cold surgery' procedure, but for the traumatic amputee, injury and operation may occur within hours of each other. The psychological support required will vary and so the demands on the nurse will depend on each individual's needs. Nurses are the only professional group readily at hand to the patients 24 hours a day and so it is to the nurses, especially in the early stages, that the patients and their relatives will turn for support and reassurance.

Nursing such patients on wards that are experienced in the care of amputation and diabetes, for example, will improve the rehabilitative care of these patients and avoid nurses feeling they have inadequate expertise and facilities, which are a main failure in the care they provide. Some, however, feel that nursing amputees throughout their operation and rehabilitative phases on an acute surgical ward is not ideal as their care tends to be superseded by the more immediate needs of the post-operative patients (Stewart, 1985). Amputee patients need nursing support in this phase too but once having recovered from the operation and become medically fit, the amputees programmed day is chiefly with other members of the multidisciplinary clinical team, mainly the physiotherapist and occupational therapist. Patients will therefore become less dependent on the nurse as time progresses and the need for drugs, dressing changes and help with functional activities on the ward, diminishes.

Some feel that nursing vascular amputees on vascular surgery wards is not good for patients undergoing vascular reconstruction, and that vascular, traumatic and oncology amputees should return to rehabilitative wards for their rehabilitation phase. Whenever this is possible and care can be continued by the same clinical team, which includes the operating surgeon, this is desirable. Sadly this is rarely possible in the UK and with the current financial situation there are few plans for new rehabilitation wards. Therefore, patients who have had surgical procedures that leave them disabled to a greater or lesser degree are nursed on the same ward. Amputees on acute surgical wards are therefore like orthopaedic patients who have had a hip or knee replacement on acute orthopaedic wards, cancer patients who have had colostomies on acute surgical wards or medical patients who have a stroke on an acute medical ward. All require a programme of care that is well planned by experts and well co-ordinated to ensure that discharge and return to the local community is swift, well organized and successful.

In the pre-operative stage, concurrent diseases will be investigated and treated appropriately. These may include treatment of the patient's diabetes, hypertension, cardiac and respiratory condition, infection, dehydration, malignancy, fractures and malnutrition. For example, subclinical protein and calorie malnutrition has been identified in as many as 50% of medical and surgical patients (Dickhaut *et al.*, 1984). Socio-economic deprivation, disease, injury and various treatments may affect the patient's nutritional status by impairing his ability to eat or absorb nutrients, or both, and by increasing the metabolic rate. Protein malnutrition has been found to be responsible for increasing mortality and post-operative morbidity, including impaired healing and an increase in wound infections (Dickhaut *et al.*, 1984). Correcting existing nutritional deficiencies prior to amputation may favourably affect healing, which is dependent upon the nutritional status of the patient as well as tissue blood supply, surgical skills, wound management. The haemoglobin level of the patient may also require treatment. Bailey *et al.* (1979) found that levels greater than 13.0 g/dl led to failed amputations and therefore promoted haemoglobin levels at the lower end of the generally accepted normal range for successful surgical results.

Pain control

For the patient already in hospital, analgesic cover will have begun, but for the newly admitted patient early assessment and treatment of pain is very important. This may be by the hospital team of doctors or the pain control team. In either case treatment must be aimed at keeping the patient's pain well under control constantly rather than administering 'top-up' injections when tablets taken regularly fail to work. Pain that is well controlled will help prepare the patient for the operation by allowing periods of rest and sleep, which will increase the desire for eating and mobilizing as appropriate.

There are three aspects of pain: the physical, the social and environmental and the psychological. In establishing the physical aspects the following points should be investigated: the onset, the site of the pain, the description of the pain with cultural and ethnic considerations, the factors which affect the pain, any previous treatment and previous pain history. Social and environmental factors include the home, family, housing and work situation and the patient's interests. Psychological aspects include anxiety and depression, the patient's mood and personality.

There are different types of pain which also need to be established. They are bone, visceral or nerve, all of which may also have a central component (Latham, 1989, personal communication). Bone pain (due to cutting the periosteum) is described as a deep ache like toothache. Vascular pain, due to an inadequate blood supply and muscle spasm is described as a throbbing or biting pain. Nerve pain is generally described as a sharp, shooting type of pain (Mensch and Ellis, 1987). Following amputation patients will always suffer from 'wound pain'. This may be superficial and local, due to surgery or, more seriously, a deep pain which is generally due to infection and needs to be investigated to ensure early treatment and avoid stump breakdown.

Drugs that are commonly used for the amputee are the non-steroidal, anti-inflammatory (NSAID), narcotic agonists and the narcotic agonist–antagonist groups. The NSAID drugs have a vascular anti-inflammatory component and aspirin and benorylate are commonly prescribed as they inhibit prostaglandin release. The narcotic agonists act on the perception of pain by the brain and stimulate the opiate receptors. In the moderate group codeine phosphate and dihydrocodeine (DF118) are commonly prescribed. In the more potent group morphine sulphate, as tablets (MST), and diamorphine are used. Palfium is also in this group and is commonly used as a 'pain break' for dressing changes for example, having an effect which lasts for 1–2 hours. The narcotic agonist–antagonist group is becoming more popular. They act as narcotic agonists and include Temgesic and Fortral. They should not, however, be used with agonist analgesics, for example those previously described. Nerve-type pain is often treated with amitriptyline and Motival is successfully used for phantom pain (Latham, 1989, personal communication). If the patient complains of a persistent pain that is difficult to relieve 24–72 hours post-operatively, this is likely to be due to haematoma formation and if this is not evacuated the increased tension will cause devitalized tissue and wound breakdown. An increased pulse rate and slight rise in temperature is also associated with this condition.

The majority of patients about to undergo amputation have tissue infections (which is common when blood supply is poor), for which suitable antibiotic treatment is also necessary. These antibiotics include those against both anaerobic and aerobic organisms, for example penicillin or a broad spectrum cephalosporin and metronidazole. The skin of the thigh is often colonized with bacteria from the alimentary canal and antibiotic treatment is necessary to prevent infections occurring, especially at the above-knee level of amputation (Browse, 1974). Gas gangrene is always a possibility and antibiotics such as penicillin and ampicillin are commonly used. The greatest cover for infection is achieved by giving systemic antibiotics less than 3 hours pre-operatively. Topical agents have not been found to be of value. If at the end of the first week the patient complains of a throbbing pain with a rise in temperature, pulse and respiratory rate, an infected wound should be considered. The wound should be inspected and pus released and suitable antibiotic treatment given following swab and culture results.

The diabetic patient must be actively investigated in this pre-operative period and the operative management of the diabetes planned. This may include the use of insulin pumps post-operatively. Other necessary investigations are discussed in Chapter 5.

During this phase the patient's social and physical needs will be assessed by the nurses, medical social worker and therapists. This information is essential for the most suitable level of amputation to be performed for each individual patient. Such details may be recorded on the nurse's care plan, or the physiotherapist's amputee assessment form (see Chapter 7). The patient who is medically fit and physically mobile, without fixed flexion contractures of the hip or knee, who is well motivated and living with or near a caring family or friends, should accept amputation, mobilize well and become a prosthetic wearer. For such a patient, the surgeon should aim for the most distal amputation that will heal, generally at the below-knee level. For the medically and physically less fit patient who has had a previous amputation and has other medical complications (e.g. hemiplegia), with few if any caring family members or friends and who is poorly motivated, the prospect of becoming a prosthetic user is slim and an amputation that will be useful in a wheelchair should be planned. To ensure successful practice, each patient must be assessed by the multidisciplinary clinical team in this pre-operative phase and the findings discussed with the surgeon so that the most suitable amputation level for the individual, that will heal primarily is chosen. In the past, the choice of level selection was made

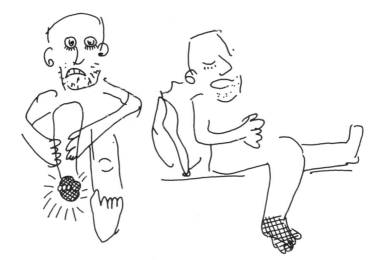

Figure 7.1 Typical positions adopted by the ischaemic patient.

by the surgeon alone but this is not regarded as good modern practice today. Level selection can be a very difficult decision for the surgeon to make but with findings, comments and support from all the other team members the decision is easier to make.

Amputation is not a 'small operation' and the patients must be adequately assessed before it is carried out (Browse, 1974). Vascular amputees often develop flexion contractures of the hip and knee in the weeks preceding amputation as they try to relieve the pain by either rubbing the foot or by hanging the leg out of the bed. Both aim to increase the blood supply to the ischaemic areas and cooling the leg by hanging it out of the bed reduces the demand by the tissues for oxygenated blood (Figure 7.1).

Good pain control is essential at this stage to allow a normal position to be resumed and also to allow physiotherapy, where necessary, to be performed.

OPERATIVE PHASE

There are two aspects in the operative phase in which ward personnel are directly involved: pre-medication and preparation of the limb for surgery.

Pre-medication

Pre-medication is given to patients before operation as both a sedative and an antisialogogue. The doses are assessed by the anaesthetist, taking into account the patient's weight, age and general condition. Often a sedative is prescribed the evening before surgery and 'nil by mouth' is taken after midnight (Haines, 1977). If the operation is planned for late in the day then 'nil by mouth' operates for 4 hours prior to surgery. This especially applies in the case of elderly and young patients who are unable to starve for long periods. Often today, spinal anaesthesia is used for amputations in the elderly as they are systemically less 'traumatic' for the patient. Patients are generally nursed flat (supine) for 12 hours following the spinal injection. This method is preferred by surgeons and nurses alike as it allows early oral fluid intake post-operatively (Mann and Bisset, 1983). Good medical care, light anaesthesia and a short operating time with the least amount of blood loss all contribute to the success of surgery in the aged and maintain low morbidity and mortality results.

Limb preparation

Patients who have infections pre-operatively are more likely to have infections post-operatively. Preparation of the leg for surgery is therefore an important procedure. The skin is painted with Povidone Iodine (Betadine) 30 minutes before surgery, which helps to reduce the spore count and the bacterial population of the skin (Tripes and Pollack, 1981). Painting should be extensive and the infected foot or leg wrapped in a plastic dressing again to prevent infection spreading (Murdoch, 1977). Shaving of the limb should be avoided, especially in the diabetic, as the small cuts only serve to add potential skin areas for infection (Westaby and White, 1985). Elderly patients having above-knee amputations are generally catheterized pre-operatively to prevent urinary contamination of the stump dressing. Perineal pads worn pre- and post-operatively also help to reduce the incidence of wound infection from clostridal spores (Robinson, 1976). The longer a patient is in hospital pre-operatively and the longer his operation, the more likely he is to develop a wound infection (Westaby and White, 1985).

IMMEDIATE POST-OPERATIVE PHASE

In the immediate post-operative phase, the vital signs of pulse, blood pressure, temperature and respiratory rate are routinely recorded, as is bleeding or drainage from the stump. Biochemistry results, metabolic and electrolytic, are routinely monitored and drugs such as antibiotics and analgesia are given regularly. Infection between the first and third post-operative day is generally due to *Clostridium welchi*; between the second and third day, due to *Streptococcus*; between the third and fifth day, due to *Staphylococcus*; and after five or more days, due to gram negative rods or mixed organisms.

It is also important that the sleep pattern be noted to ensure that the patient is receiving adequate sleep at night to cope with his demanding physical programme during the day. The nursing staff ensure that the patient's bed is firm to prevent flexion contractures developing and to make transfers, especially for the bilateral amputee, easier to perform. Bed cradles, ripple mattresses, sheep skin bootees and monkey poles may also be used as aids to mobility or to prevent pressure areas developing. Early mobilization and sitting out of bed are encouraged from the second post-operative day, ensuring that the below-knee stump is well supported in a level position. It is important that the nurse responds normally to the amputated leg and never shows any signs of physical avoidance in the care activities (Stewart, 1985). Trans-cutaneous nerve stimulation (TNS) given at a low frequency has also been found to reduce pain (Latham, 1987) and to help heal stumps by acting as a vasodilator (Finsen *et al.*, 1988).

Contractures develop due to either a muscle imbalance due to surgical division of the muscles acting around a joint, or to previous disease and poor postural habit over a long period of time. Lying prone for one to three half-hour periods a day has been advocated in the past as a way of preventing flexion contractures at the hip and knee. With good surgery, analgesic cover and an active exercise programme, prone lying is unnecessary. The majority of today's amputees, the elderly, diabetic, obese and those with respiratory or cardiac conditions, are both unable to tolerate lying prone and will resist resting in this position. Resting on the top of the bed in a supine position that keeps the hip and knee flat for periods in the day will serve two purposes. It will stop the patient becoming 'chair shaped' in flexion and rest him before more rehabilitative activities take place.

In the early post-operative days it will be beneficial for the patients to be exposed to prostheses on an informal basis. This helps to prepare them and their relatives for the future. If the patient does become a prosthetic wearer it is the nurse's role to encourage him to keep trying to use and accept the prosthesis (Stewart, 1985). The nurse can also help by encouraging the patient to exercise and by providing opportunities for the patient to do things for him-/herself and become independent on the ward. Liaison with the therapy staff through weekly team meetings is vital for the patient's maximum potential to be reached.

Hopping with crutches was commonly practised with staff walking near the patient 'lest he slips' (Browse, 1974). Practice today is to keep elderly patients in a wheelchair until they are walking on a prosthesis to avoid falls and the stump becoming oedematous by being held dependent. Falls should be avoided at all costs in the early stages before healing has occurred. For the younger, traumatic amputee whose reflexes are intact, hopping with crutches will be taught. Patients are, however, taught to hop as a functional activity, for example getting to the toilet when the prosthesis is not being worn or for the functional needs of the non-walker.

In the early post-operative period, in the UK a Department of Health AOF3 form is sent to the local Disablement Services or Prosthetic Centre for a prosthetic assessment appointment. When attending for the appointment the patient takes hospital medical notes and information regarding the physical, psychological and social situation, so that the most suitable prosthesis is prescribed. Also in the first week or two post-operatively, an early home visit by two team members (without the patient) to the patient's home should be arranged to meet the family and neighbours and to assess the housing, equipment and social service requirements that will be necessary for return to the community. Contacts with the district nurse by the hospital nurses, if this is appropriate, will also be made early in the patient's hospitalization period to ensure adequate and continued care is given on the patient's discharge. The possibility for weekend leave will also be assessed on the early home visit so that the rehabilitative phase is split up and that contacts at home and in the community are maintained. This ensures the patient does not become too hospitalized.

DRESSING TECHNIQUES

When considering a post-operative dressing method for the amputee stump, a number of factors need to be taken into consideration. These are:

1. protection of the wound from bacterial infection;
2. control or prevention of oedema;
3. support and protection of the wound from local physical trauma;
4. the ease and training required to use the technique;
5. the speed and frequency of its application; and
6. the ease of applying an early walking aid or weight bearing as required.

There are three main methods used today and the choice of technique is very dependent on local factors such as the specialized staff required, patient population, nurse staffing levels and rehabilitation routines. The stump environment chosen must be one that is least likely to harm the patient and possibly provide some control of oedema (Murdoch, 1983). The three main methods are soft dressings, semi-rigid dressings and rigid dressings.

Soft dressing techniques

Bandages

Soft dressings, although thought to be outdated by some, remain a popular form of post-operative dressing technique for the amputee

(Mensch and Ellis, 1987). Bandages are inexpensive and readily available in hospital and some nurses are trained in their application. Sustained pressures greater than 15 mmHg have been found to decrease flow (Spiro *et al.*, 1980) and sustained pressures greater than 25 mmHg have been found to be potentially harmful (Müller and Vetter, 1954). Intercapillary pressure varies with dependency therefore the ideal bandage should provide graded pressure that is maximal at the most distal point and decreases proximally (Isherwood *et al.*, 1975).

The pressure that is applied is inversely proportional to the radius of curvature of the limb. Pressures greater than 15–20 mmHg applied to the popliteal fossa have been found to cause a tourniquet effect even when the whole limb is wrapped (Hosni *et al.*, 1968) and it has been recommended that no dressing with a pressure greater than 10 mmHg should be left overnight (Johnson, 1972). Isherwood compared pressures under amputee dressings that had been applied by staff skilled in bandage application (nurses and physiotherapists) with unskilled bandagers (patients and relatives). The majority of readings were found to be up to 50 mmHg but pressures up to 140 mmHg by skilled and 170 mmHg by unskilled operators were recorded. Elastic bandages can therefore be potentially dangerous and detrimental to the blood flow in a limb especially when applied by unskilled operators.

Soft dressings remain popular, and most surgeons use gauze, cotton wool and crepe bandages immediately post-operatively (Browse, 1974). Advantages are that they are inexpensive, readily available, quick to apply and they make frequent observations of the wound possible. The disadvantages are that their frequent changes disturbs healing tissue, oedema is allowed to form and the tension applied cannot be accurately controlled which can lead to pain. Some authors feel that joint contractures are more likely to develop and that movement of the knee may hinder the suture line from healing with this type of dressing (Mensch and Ellis, 1987). *Clostridia* have been found in non-sterile bandages so it is important to maintain a sterile barrier between the unhealed wound and the bandage (Pearson *et al.*, 1980). The use of sticky tape should be avoided with the vascular patient, as blistering, subsequent infection and necrosis can occur.

Cylindrical soft dressings

A light elastic, cylindrical dressing, for example Seton's Tubifast, may be used over a wool pad once the theatre crepe dressing is rolled down and the redivac suction drains removed (Figure 7.2). Tubifast is applied with a Seton's applicator and is changed daily. No tape is required to

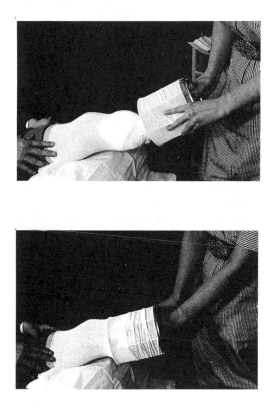

Figure 7.2 Application of Seton's Tubifast.

hold the dressing on, as the below-knee dressing is applied well over the knee joint and for the above knee, up into the groin. Oedema is controlled, the wounds heal, joint contractures do not develop as exercising starts on the first post-operative day and the use of an early walking aid is possible from approximately the seventh post-operative day.

The Puddifoot dressing

The Puddifoot soft dressing technique was first described in 1973. Following surgery, a sterile gauze dressing is applied over the wound and a cotton sock over the whole stump. A strip of foam the width of the stump is placed over the stump in an anteroposterior direction and the lateral sections are also filled with foam. Seton's Tubigrip, a cylindrical dressing closed at one end, is then applied over the stump and a waist belt is used for the above-knee stump so that the dressing does not roll down. Pressure measurements under such a dressing have been recorded and almost half of the readings were found to be below 11 mmHg which would have little effect on oedema control (Puddifoot *et al.*, 1973).

Shrinker socks

Shrinker socks (e.g. Truform USA, Jobst, Juzo-Varin) are becoming increasingly popular for use with the elderly vascular amputee patient for their ease of application (Nirula, 1986). The stump length and circumference measurements are taken and the appropriate sock size used. Such socks have been found to be effective in reducing oedema and residual stump volume in the well-healed stump (Manella, 1981). Caution should be taken when used on the unhealed stump, especially a vascular stump when a larger size than measured is used. Application is made easier with the use of a Seton's metal applicator.

Semi-rigid dressing techniques

There are two types of semi-rigid dressings used for the amputee stump, the Unna paste dressing and pneumatic dressings.

Unna paste technique

Unna paste is composed of zinc oxide, glycerine, gelatin and water. The zinc oxide has a soothing and protective effect on the skin, possibly acting as an astringent, the gelatin acts as a mechanical, protective agent giving a suitable consistence for application, the glycerine acts as a humectant keeping the mixture moist and preventing evaporation taking place too quickly and the wound drying out and the water acts as a dilutant making the mixture easier to apply.

The dressing is applied in the operating theatre. A sterile gauze dressing covers the wound and a gauze bandage impregnated with Unna paste covers the stump. Felt pads are then positioned to protect pressure-sensitive areas and a second Unna bandage is applied with diagonal turns. With the below-knee stumps, the bandage is applied to the mid-thigh and for the above-knee stumps, a hip spica may be included. The stump position is carefully monitored for the 12–24 hours it takes to dry to ensure no flexion contracture develops.

The advantages of this dressing are that it is lightweight, soft and, because of its total contact nature, maintains the shape of the stump and controls oedema. It allows some freedom of movement and can be kept in place for several days before it is changed (Holliday, 1981). It is also said to promote primary healing (Mensch and Ellis, 1987).

Pneumatic dressings

Two types of pneumatic dressing techniques are available, the air splint and controlled environment treatment.

The air splint. The air splint was originally used in emergency situations to stabilize fractures or limb injuries. In the early 1970s it was used for the amputee stump (Little, 1971). Air splints can be supplied in the form of a boot (Jobst Postop air boot) or with a metal frame (Jobst Softstem). The air splints are sterilized and made of clear plastic with a front zipper for ease of application. They are applied in the operating theatre over a sterile gauze dressing and possibly a wool pad, stump sock and relief pads made of felt, that are held in place by a surgical adhesive spray (Mensch and Ellis 1987). Dressings are changed at 3, 5, 7 and 10 days when an alternative compression dressing may be used (Holliday, 1981). Pressures of 27 mmHg have been said to be well tolerated for the 10 day period (Sher and Liebman, 1982) but other authors suggest that lower pressures may have less detrimental effects on a healing stump (Hosni *et al.*, 1968; Johnson, 1972; Spiro *et al.*, 1980).

By using pneumatic devices and increasing the pressure, weight bearing has been possible (Little, 1971). With the air boot, increasing the pressure to 45–50 mmHg allows weight bearing for short periods with no adverse effects (Holliday, 1981). However, as the pressure inside the splint increases as it takes the patient's weight, the suspension tends to reduce as the device becomes compressed and moves. This is most noticeable with the above-knee amputee (Monga *et al.*, 1985).

The Jobst 'Softstem' prosthesis with an aluminium external support has been used from the fifth to seventh post-operative day with pressures of 40 mmHg (Kerstein, 1985) and the Vessa Pneumatic Postamputation Mobility Aid (Ppam aid) is started on the seventh post-operative day with pressures of 40 mmHg (Redhead *et al.*, 1978) (see Chapter 8).

The advantages of the air splint are that it is easy to apply, it is readily available and can be used by relatively unskilled personnel and that it gives uniform pressure to the stump. It has been found to speed up stump maturation, decrease the deterioration of postural reflexes and shorten the time between surgery and prosthetic fitting (Pollack and Kerstein, 1985). It is easy to remove to check the wound, protects the stump from local trauma, has been found to help reduce oedema and pain (Sher and Liebman, 1982) and does not interfere with the eventual gait pattern of the below-knee amputee (Bonner and Green, 1982). Its disadvantages are that the stump perspires, there can be air leakage though never rapid, and that it is a bulky 'dressing' which reduces bed and knee mobility. The device holds the above-knee stump in slight flexion which encourages a flexion contracture to develop and it is bulky and clumsy for the patient when he is sitting in a wheelchair (Mensch and Ellis, 1987).

Controlled environment treatment. Controlled environment treatment (CET) was developed at Biomechanical Research and Development Unit, London, as a wound management system for the amputee stump (Redhead and Snowdon, 1978). The bare limb is placed in a transparent plastic film bag and a variable, cyclic, pressurized gaseous environment surrounds the limb providing direct pressure. The system is used 24 hours a day for an average of 10 days. In some centres it is used for up to 21 days. The advantages of the system are that it protects the wound from bacterial contamination, and that the low relative humidity around the stump maintains the skin in a dry state, therefore reducing bacterial levels. The pressure used to control oedema is uniform, therefore there is no tourniquet effect and the required temperature can be set. It is simple to set up, wound and muscle activity are clearly visible and knee flexion to approximately 60 degrees is possible (Kegel, 1976).

The equipment is, however, initially expensive and noisy in use and the patient tends to be bed or ward bound for the 10 day period. Care has to be taken to avoid pressure sores by encouraging the patient to move about the bed and exercising to prevent hip and knee flexion contractures. Although some authors feel it has advantages over rigid techniques (Kegel, 1976) as more muscle groups can be exercised early, other authors feel it has no advantages over a rigid method (Ruckley *et al.*, 1986) and others recommend its use when there is a possibility of complications in the healing of wounds, either surgical or traumatic (Burgess, 1978).

Rigid dressing techniques

The rigid dressing technique was originated by Berlemont of France in 1961, who used a plaster of Paris (POP) cast over the amputation stump which incorporated a temporary prosthesis (Berlemont *et al.*, 1969). Weiss of Poland modified the technique with his experience of stump revisions of traumatic amputations after the Second World War (Weiss, 1966) and the technique became popularized in the USA by Burgess. Although a rigid dressing of POP remains popular in the USA, the early prosthetic gait unit attachment has been abandoned in many centres. POP dressings are also used in amputee centres in the UK that are run in conjunction with orthopaedic departments.

The rigid dressing is applied in the operating theatre following amputation. The wound is covered with a sterile gauze or silicone-impregnated dressing, fluffed gauze and an elastic stump sock which is held in place by adhesive surgical spray. Pressure-sensitive areas are relieved by sterilized precut felt pads and finally an elasticated POP bandage is applied ensuring that the cast conforms well to the stump shape (Murdoch, 1983; Mensch and Ellis, 1987). The cast takes 24 hours to dry and close observations have to be kept during this time by trained personnel to ensure that the dressing is not too tight. The patient is nursed in bed during this period and the cast supported throughout its length. The cast remains on for approximately 10–14 days but early cast changes may be indicated if it loosens, rotates or becomes excessively tight. If it becomes damaged or the patient experiences severe pain or feels a pressure area, perhaps from a crease in the sock or POP bandage, it will also be changed. If the patient becomes febrile, toxic or the cast develops an odour, again it will be changed. Casts are usually changed at 5 days (Kraker *et al.*, 1986).

The advantages of the rigid dressing are that it controls post-operative stump oedema by maintaining an even pressure and gives protection to the stump. It provides tissue support and therefore reduces pain and discomfort and allows for early ambulation without interfering with the wound site (Mensch and Ellis, 1987). This dressing method must, however, be applied by trained personnel who are familiar with POP techniques and this often includes the prosthetist. Ward staff must be well informed of the signs of early complications and the appropriate action that should be taken. Wound inspection is not easily possible but some feel that this is an advantage as the healing process is not disturbed. POP may be harmful when used with the senile patient, those who suffer with mental confusion, severe cardiac or neurological disability and is not thought to be helpful for those patients who have a short life expectancy (Kane and Pollack, 1980). Ambulation starts at approximately 5–12 days post-operatively with the application of the prosthetic gait attachment (Kraker *et al.*, 1986).

Immediate post-operative fitting

By adding a prosthetic attachment and foot onto a rigid dressing, weight bearing is allowed to take place as early as 24 hours post-operatively. However, many centres have abandoned the use of immediate post-operative fitting due to a high incidence of wound complications, delayed wound healing and high re-amputation rates (Mooney *et al.*, 1971).

A study in 1980 compared the use of rigid and soft dressing techniques and found that hospital time, morbidity, mortality and functional recovery were similar. However, the amount of narcotics taken for pain was higher in the rigid dressing group (Kane and Pollack, 1980).

PHANTOM SENSATION AND PHANTOM PAIN

Phantom pain was first described by Ambrose Paré in the sixteenth century and later by Weir Mitchell during the American Civil War (Miles, 1989). It can be described as a painful sensation that feels as though it is emanating from the amputated portion of the limb. Virtually all amputees have various types of persistent phantom sensation that may be painful (Sherman, 1980). The abnormal sensation may range from slight tingling or numbness to severe tearing or crushing pain (Troop and Wood, 1982). Phantom pain should not, however, be confused with stump pain which has a different location to phantom pain.

Phantom sensation or phantom limb is commonly experienced following amputation. An image of the absent limb is produced in the cerebral cortex through stimulation of the sensory nerve endings in the amputated stump. This is, however, not possible with the congenital limb absence cases as the body image in the cerebral cortex has never been complete. Telescoping, or the reducing of the image of the leg in the brain, is felt for some time. The feet and toes, especially the big toe, are often the last to fade. This is, however, rare with Syme or partial foot amputation (Dickhaut *et al.*, 1984). Phantom limb sensation is an asset to the patient when he starts limb wearing as he feels he is moving his own leg rather than a prosthesis. All patients and relatives should be warned of this pre-operatively.

Pain is very personal and the patient's emotional state may influence the degree of phantom pain that he is experiencing. Other causes of stump pain, for example scars and neuroma, may need surgical attention. No single treatment is satisfactory for all cases of phantom pain. A review of 43 different treatments used in the treatment of this condition were divided into two main groups: those that worked by physically altering the signals from the stump to the brain, and those that altered the interpretation of the 'pain' signals. The first group can be subdivided into those treatments that supplement the signal, for example percussion, TNS, relaxation, exercise, warm baths, massage, ultrasound or acupuncture, and those treatments that remove some of the incoming signals, for example surgery to the stump, procaine blocks, sympathectomy, trigger point elimination and central nerve blocks. The second group can be subdivided into three groups: those treatments that physically alter the interpretative centre of the brain, treatments using chemical methods to alter the interpretation of pain stimuli and treatments using behavioural methods of altering the interpretation of 'pain' signals. Other treatments tried have included vitamin B_{12} therapy, radiation, thermography and magnetotherapy. It was found that treatments were ineffective at the one year follow-up. Most treatments worked temporarily for a third of the patients treated. This figure is similar to that found in other studies on surgical patients where the short-term 'cure' rate was 35%. It is therefore tempting to say that the cure is due to the placebo effect (Sherman, 1980).

Parkes (1973) wrote that the personality of the patient experiencing phantom pain was rigid and compulsively self-reliant which is completely different from the personalities of placebo responders who are anxious, dependent, self-centred and emotional. It must therefore be presumed that treatments are likely to be effective only for some patients and some aetiologies.

Renström (1987) interviewed 66 patients to determine the nature, timing and location of their pain. The character of the pain was described as flashing (33%), cramp (5.6%), itching and flashing (7.4%), itching (5.6%) and burning (3.7%). A third of the patients experienced the pain daily, 26% weekly, 7.4% monthly and 22% seldom. For the majority it only lasted seconds (27.7%) or minutes (35%) but some experienced it for hours (14.8%) or days (5.6%). The location of the pain was chiefly in toes (37%) or toes and foot (61%). Phantom pain in the whole amputated part was experienced by 18.5% of patients.

REFERENCES

Bailey, M.J., Johnston, C.L.W., Yates, C.J.P., Somerville, P.G. and Dormandy, J.A. (1979) Preoperative haemoglobin as predictor of outcome of diabetic amputations. *Lancet*, **i**, 168–170.

Berlemont, M., Weber, R. and Willot, J.P. (1969) Ten years of experience with the immediate application of prosthetic devices to amputees of the lower extremities on the operative room table. *Prosthet Int.*, **3**, 8–18.

Bonner, F.J. and Green, R.F. (1982) Pneumatic airleg prosthesis: Report of 200 cases. *Arch. Phys. Med. Rehabil.*, **63**, 383–385.

Browse, N.L. (1974) Amputation of the lower limb. *Nursing Mirror*, 7 June, 63–65.

Burgess, E.M. (1978) Wound healing after amputation: effect of controlled environment treatment. *J. Bone Joint Surg.*, **60**, 245–246.

Dickhaut, S.C., De Lee, J.C. and Page, C.P. (1984) Nutritional status: importance in predicting wound healing after amputation. *J. Bone Joint Surg.*, **66A**, 71–75.

Finsen, V., Persen, L., Løvlien, M., Veslegaard, E.K., Simensis, M., Gasvann, A.K. and Benum, P. (1988) Transcutaneous electrical nerve stimulation after major amputation. *J. Bone Joint Surg.*, **70B**, 109–112.

Haines, A.M. (1977) Anaesthesia in the elderly, in *Geriatric Orthopaedics* (ed. M. Devas), Academic Press, New York, pp. 31–38.

Holliday, P.J. (1981) Early postoperative care of the amputee, in *Amputation Surgery and Rehabilitation – the Toronto Experience*, Churchill Livingstone, Edinburgh, pp. 217–232.

Hosni, E.A., Ximenes, J.O.C. and Hamilton, F.G. (1968) Pressure bandaging of the lower extremity. *JAMA*, **206**, 2715–2718.

Isherwood, P.A., Robertson, J.C. and Rossi, A. (1975) Pressure measurements beneath below-knee amputation stump bandages: elastic bandaging, the Puddifoot dressing and a pneumatic bandaging technique compared. *Br. J. Surg.*, **62**, 982–986.

Johnson, H.D. (1972) Mechanics of elastic bandaging (correspondence). *Br. Med. J.*, **3**, 767–768.

Kane, T.J. and Pollack, E.W. (1980) The rigid versus soft post-operative dressing controversy: a controlled study in vascular below-knee amputees. *Am. Surgeon*, April, 244–247.

Kegel, B. (1976) Controlled environment treatment (CET) for patients with below-knee amputations. *Phys. Ther.*, **56**, 1366–1371.

Kerstein, M.D. (1985) An improved modality in lower extremity amputee rehabilitation. *Orthopaedics*, **8**, 207–209.

Kraker, D., Pinzur, M.S., Daley, R. and Osterman, H. (1986) Early post surgical prosthetic fitting with a prefabricated plastic limb. *Orthopaedics*, **9**, 989–992.

Latham, J. (1987) Transcutaneous nerve stimulation. *The Professional Nurse*, February, 133–135.

Little, J.M. (1971) A pneumatic weight-bearing temporary prosthesis for below-knee amputees. *Lancet*, **i**, 271–272.

Manella, K.J. (1981) Comparing the effectiveness of elastic bandages to shrinker socks for lower extremity amputees. *Phys. Ther.*, **61**, 334–337.

Mann, R.A.M. and Bisset, W.I.K. (1983) Anaesthesia for lower limb amputation. *Anaesthesia*, **38**, 1185–1191.

Mensch, G. and Ellis, P.M. (1987) Preoperative and postoperative care and the responsibility of the physical therapist, in *Physical Therapy Management of Lower Extremity Amputations*, Heinemann Physiotherapy, London, pp. 45–96.

Miles, J. (1989) Phantom limb pain, in *Step Forward NALD*, spring 1989, issue 14.

Monga, T.N., Symington, D.C., Lowe, P. and Elkin, N. (1985) Load bearing and suspension characteristics of airsplint as a temporary prosthesis. *Prosthet. Orthot. Int.*, **9**, 100–104.

Mooney, V., Harvey, J.P., McBride, E. and Snelson, R. (1971) Comparison of post-operative stump management: plaster vs. soft dressings. *J. Bone Joint Surg.*, **53A**, 241–249.

Müller, E.A. and Vetter, K. (1954) The effect of pressure loads upon blood supply to the skin. *Arbeitsphysiologie*, **15**, 295–304.

Murdoch, G. (1977) Amputation surgery in the lower extremity. *Prosthet. Orthot. Int.*, **1**, 72–83.

Murdoch, G. (1983) The post-operative environment of the amputation stump. *Prosthet. Orthot. Int.*, **7**, 75–78.

Nirula, H.C. (1986) Clinical evaluation of Juzo stump compression supports. ALAC Medical Officers AGM.

Parkes, C. (1973) Factors determining the persistence of phantom pain in the amputee. *J. Psychosomatic Res.*, **17**, 97–108.

Pearson, R.D., Valenti, W.M. and Steigbigel, R.T. (1980) *Clostridium perfringens* wound infection associated with elastic bandages. *JAMA*, **244**, 1128–1130.

Pollack, C.V. and Kerstein, M.D. (1985) Prevention of post operative complications in the lower extremity amputee. *J. Cardiovasc. Surg.*, **26**, 287–290.

Puddifoot, P.C., Weaver, P.C. and Marshall, S.A. (1973) A method of supportive bandaging for amputation stumps. *Br. J. Surg.*, **60**, 729–731.

Redhead, R.G. and Snowdon, C. (1978) A new approach to the management of wounds of the extremities: controlled environment treatment and its derivatives. *Prosthet. Orthot. Int.*, **2**, 148–156.

Redhead, R.G., Davis, B.C., Robinson, K.P. and Vitali, M. (1978) Post-amputation pneumatic walking aid. *Br. J. Surg.*, **65**, 611–612.

Renström, P. (1981) Below knee amputees at an amputee training centre, in *The Below Knee Amputee*, University of Göteborg, Sweden, pp. 31–44.

Robinson, K.P. (1976) Long posterior flap amputation in geriatric patients with ischaemic disease. *Ann. R. Coll. Surg. (Eng.)*, **58**, 440–451.

Ruckley, C.V., Rae, A. and Prescott, R.J. (1986) Controlled environment unit in the care of the below-knee amputation stump. *Br. J. Surg.*, **73**, 11–13.

Sher, M.H. and Liebman, P. (1982) The air splint: a method of managing below-knee amputations. *J. Cardiovas. Surg.*, **23**, 407–410.

Sherman, R.A. (1980) Published treatments of phantom limb pain. *Am. J. Phys. Med.*, **59**, 232–244.

Spiro, M., Roberts, V.C. and Richardson, J.B. (1980) The effect of externally applied pressure on femoral vein blood flow. *Br. Med. J.*, **1**, 719–723.

Stewart, A. (1985) Diabetes and amputation at 73. *Nursing Times*, 24 July, 39–41.

Tripes, D. and Pollack, E.W. (1981) Risk factors in healing of below knee amputations. *Am. J. Surg.*, **141**, 718–720.

Troop, I.M. and Wood, M.A. (1982) The stump – function and associated problems, in *Total Care of the Lower Limb Amputee*, Pitman Books, New York, pp.76–79.

Weiss, M. (1966) The prosthesis on the operating table from the neurophysio-logical point of view. Report of the Workshop Panel in Lower Extremity Prosthetics Fitting, Committee on Prosthetics Research and Development, National Academy of Science Meeting, 6–9 February 1966.

Westaby, S. and White, S. (1985) Wound infection, in *Wound Care* (ed. S. Westaby.), Heinemann Medical Books, London.

8

The rehabilitation process

INTRODUCTION

The rehabilitation process following amputation is generally regarded as retraining in physical, functional and social activities and the activities are carried out under the guidance of the occupational therapist and physiotherapist. Physical training is predominantly carried out by the physiotherapist (PT) and functional and social training by the occupational therapist (OT). There are areas of overlap where in one locality the activity may be carried out by the OT and in another area it may be carried out by the PT. The variations are due in general to the local environment, staffing, personalities, interest and a good team approach. In a good team approach situation, as discussed in Chapter 6, the flexibility and overlap of roles and activities should be totally acceptable to all members of the team.

This chapter covers the stages of the rehabilitation process highlighting the roles of each therapist. (As the majority of therapists in the west are female and the majority of amputees are male, 'she' and 'he' will be used throughout for simplicity.)

THE PROFESSIONALS

The quality of therapy that the patient receives depends almost entirely on the quality of the therapist, her understanding of the patient and his disability, her detailed knowledge of the available therapeutic techniques, a sound knowledge of medical and surgical care, the availability and use of aids and appliances and the resettlement facilities provided by statutory and voluntary bodies. The therapist must be trained to play an important role in the assessment of the physical disability and in the instruction of techniques by which the patient can overcome or adjust to his handicap.

The therapists' role in amputee rehabilitation can be divided into three phases: the pre-operative phase, the post-operative phase, early and late, and the prosthetic phase.

THE PRE-OPERATIVE PHASE

The majority of amputations carried out today in the western world are for vascular disease. These operations are generally not carried out as emergency procedures so there is a pre-operative period which may vary from a day or two to a week or more. The therapists' role begins in this pre-operative period and should cover four areas: the introductory visit, the assessments, the discussion of results and amputation level and the operative preparation.

Introductory visit

Patients who are about to undergo amputation are often known to the staff as they may be or may have been on the ward undergoing investigations or vascular reconstructive procedures. However, for every patient, once the decision to amputate has been made, the therapists visit and introduce themselves to the patient, giving him a brief explanation of their role in the rehabilitation team.

The prospect of having an amputation comes as a shock to all patients and their families. They generally feel it is the 'end of the line' and that amputation is a negative procedure. They need reassurance that the amputation is necessary and that it is a positive step towards rehabilitation and discharge back into the community. Giving the patient and his family information about the rehabilitation procedures and some insight into the future, will help them come to terms with the operation. Realistic goals and expectations are given in such a way that the patient's motivation is not reduced and the importance of his participation in the rehabilitation process is explained to both the patient and his family.

It is generally the PT who introduces the patient and his family to the team management concept and explains the roles of the individual team members. She will liaise in this pre-operative phase with the other team members and indicate to them her findings, the amount of involvement they may expect with that individual patient and if it is necessary and essential to become involved pre-operatively. The PT has been said to be a key person in the rehabilitation of the amputee (Burgess and Alexander, 1973). This is because she spends more time with the patient than any other single member of the rehabilitation team and so develops close relationships with the patient and his family, providing him with the opportunity to express his fears, apprehensions and ambitions. An effective team approach is essential to help the patient reach his full potential and the opportunity to play a key role is one that should be accepted eagerly by the PT (Condie, 1988). For a PT to make a positive contribution as a key member and possible team co-ordinator she must be trained in this special field (Troop and Wood, 1982).

The OT's role begins whenever possible in the pre-operative period and continues during rehabilitation in hospital through to discharge. Involvement at this stage aims to reduce anxiety and to gain as much information from the patient and their family about their life-style and social life as possible to assist in the pre-operative team assessment. Many people facing an amputation are unsure how they will cope at home and they may be reassured by knowing the OT's role in helping them to regain their independence. This may also help to reduce the family's anxiety as amputation affects them also. Pre-operatively it is also useful to ask the relatives to bring in the patient's own wheelchair, if he has one, and to bring in some suitable day clothes.

The patient will be ill or toxic and very often will be unable to remember much information, therefore the reason why there is need for amputation and the information given to the patient at this time is reinforced by written information or a patient booklet (Ham and Kerfoot, 1989).

Assessments

The therapists will assess the patient's physical condition and his psychological and social state pre-operatively. It is helpful if all this information is kept together on one form. A physiotherapy assessment form is given in Appendix 8.1 as an example.

The *physical* assessment should include all aspects of the patient's health and the physical conditions that are going to affect his mobility. Examples would be a hip replacement, Dupuytren's contractures, psoriasis, poor vision or hearing or hemiplegia. It is noted if he is a smoker, if he takes any medication for a chest condition and whether he is short of breath at rest or on exertion. The patient's general muscle strength is assessed using the Medical Research Council Oxford scale

(Atkinson, 1974) and his joint ranges of motion are recorded for both upper and lower limbs. Contractures are noted, as are the patient's balance and co-ordination and his ability to transfer, for example from bed to chair. Skin condition and sensation are described and any red or broken pressure areas recorded. If the patient is walking, the distance he manages and the method he uses with or without aids are noted. If the patient has a wheelchair this is recorded and his ability to manoeuvre and transfer into it. The patient's mobility up to this admission (or if he has not been walking for some weeks or months) is also recorded and whether he was dressing, toileting or bathing without help.

During the assessment, the patient's attitude and *psychological* state are noted by the therapist. Further information from his family or carer is also useful at this time as the patient may often be in a toxic state and confused and in pain.

It is also necessary to record the patient's *social* situation as it may be relevant to the decision on the selection of the amputation level. The patient's close family, carers or friends are noted and some or all of them will be contacted in this pre-operative period. The accommodation in which the patient lives is recorded and access, stairs, steps and toilet facilities are noted as they give the team an insight into the patient's capabilities before this admission. Any help the patient requires with the cooking, laundry or shopping is also noted.

Discussion of results and selection of amputation level

Following assessment of the patient, the team meets and the results of their findings are discussed so that the most suitable level of amputation for each patient is selected. The surgeon, with the results of previous surgery or investigations, will have made a clinical assessment of the necessary level of amputation. The patient may have been assessed in a Vascular Laboratory with amputation level selection techniques such as laser Doppler or transcutaneous oximetry (Chapter 5), which indicate that a certain level of amputation is advisable. From her physical assessment, the PT will recommend a level of amputation that is physically and socially advisable for that patient and the OT will comment on her functional and social assessment. The prosthetist will give his opinions when discussions affecting prosthetic management of the patient are necessary. The nurse, social worker and clinical psychologist may add further information to the team discussions from their own assessments and observations as appropriate.

In respected centres that practise a team approach, it is only when all the team have assessed the patient and discussed their results, that the level of amputation is decided upon.

Preparation for the operation

In the pre-operative period it may be appropriate, and time may allow a visit to the gymnasium or OT department. For some patients and families it is not advisable, but for most it is recommended as they see the environment in which they will spend much of their time and meet other amputees practising their activities. Once the level of amputation has been decided upon, it may also be appropriate to show the patient a prosthesis similar to the one he may receive. If the patient is unlikely to be a prosthetic user obviously this would not be advisable. Some patients may appear lucid and well enough to absorb this information but in many cases the information is not absorbed by the patient. The visit to the gymnasium is, however, useful for the patient's family. Future amputees find it helpful to speak to other amputees, perhaps a few weeks ahead of themselves in the rehabilitation programme. If this is not possible in a hospital ward, it is often possible for the patient to be visited by an established out-patient amputee of similar age and temperament and the same projected level of amputation.

During this pre-operative phase, which may last several days, it is essential that an exercise programme is started to strengthen the patient generally and increase his mobility, keeping him walking if at all possible. It is also important to reduce or prevent flexion contractures. The amount and intensity of the treatment given by the therapists at this time will vary depending on the findings of the assessment. Pre-operative training is worth hours after the operation (Browse, 1974).

The type of anaesthetic, the use of drugs, intravenous and spinal injection, drips, pumps and epidurals must be explained to the patient and his family clearly by a member of the team. To the lay person, unfamiliar with hospitals, all of these modern procedures and practices can be terrifying if not adequately explained. Phantom sensation (Chapter 7) should also be explained at this time so that the patient is aware of the possibility of feeling such sensations post-operatively.

Loaning the patient a wheelchair and mobility aids for the bed and ward may be carried out either by the PT, OT or the nurse. (The operative preparation of the patient is discussed in Chapter 7.)

THE POST-OPERATIVE PHASE

The post-operative phase can be divided into the early and late periods. The therapist who has seen an amputation being performed has a greater understanding and is more sensitive to the patient's post-operative needs, so a visit to the operating theatre is recommended.

Early post-operative period

In the UK, the chief dressing technique used today is a soft dressing. Management of patients with plaster of Paris dressing will not be discussed here as good descriptions are given elsewhere (Mensch and Ellis, 1987). (Dressing techniques are described in Chapter 7.)

Physiotherapy

On return from the operating theatre the PT will check the patient's chest and the position of the stump. The stump should remain flat on the bed without pillows or sheets or sandbags. If for comfort a pillow is necessary under a below-knee stump then it should be placed lengthways and not crossways on the bed to minimize the tendency for the stump to become flexed.

During the first 2 days the physiotherapy sessions will be for as long as the patient can tolerate and he will receive regular drugs or an epidural infusion to keep the pain under control. The use of spinal anaesthesia reduces the complication of chest infection which is common with this group of patients. Physiotherapy is therefore directed at mobilization, muscle strengthening and the prevention of flexion contractures. It is always advisable to start the exercises on the unaffected side before the affected side. This helps to introduce the PT to the patient and accustom him to movement before moving the tender stump.

In the past all amputees were encouraged to be in the prone position for at least 30 minutes to 1 hour every day to help reduce flexion contractures. Today most of the patients are elderly, some with cardiac or respiratory conditions, and find this position uncomfortable. Patients are therefore advised to lie flat on the bed when resting to avoid the flexed position that sitting in chairs, wheelchairs and beds encourage in the early post-operative days. Good surgery, analgesia and an active exercise programme will reduce the number of flexion contractures and therefore prone lying should not be necessary in a good hospital practice today. Prone lying is, however, a good position for exercising for some patients and side lying will help to reduce and relieve pressure on the buttock region.

It is important that the movements opposite to those producing typical contractures are practised thoroughly. Chiefly these are, for the below knee, knee extension and for the above knee, hip extension. General exercises for the upper limbs and trunk are also added as appropriate. If full movements are not achieved with time spent coaxing the patient, it is advisable to ask for the analgesia to be reviewed and to treat the patient often during these early days until a full range of movement is established. Similar exercises are repeated on the second day and the patient will begin to sit out of bed. For the below-knee amputee it is important that he sits with his stump level (horizontal) to avoid oedema forming and delay healing. Orthopaedic stump boards have been used in the past, but the Rivermead (Hamilton, 1977) or the Remploy King's (Ham and Richardson, 1986) stump boards are recommended (Figure 8.1).

From approximately the third day onwards, the patient's medical condition will stabilize and the intravenous drips and suction drains will be removed. When the patient is medically fit and well enough to be

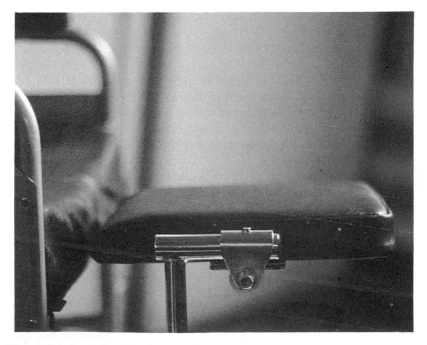

Figure 8.1 Remploy King's stump board

able to appreciate the environment of the gymnasium with other patients, treatment will continue there. The treatment sessions are organized as individual treatments and on a 'group' basis which provides both psychological and social support. Groups also help to improve the elderly patient's mental alertness and social integration (Troop and Wood, 1982). Treatment sessions should be twice a day and their length should increase as the patient becomes fitter and stronger. Patients are encouraged to start to wear day clothes at this stage.

A wide variety of exercises can be taught to improve the patient's mobility and general strength. The majority of lower limb amputees are elderly and find it difficult to learn new techniques, so a simple exercise regimen which is appropriate for these patients will be more successful. For the younger traumatic amputee, a programme that is more vigorous with greater variety will be necessary and for the young child it will be more appropriate to treat the child with the mother's assistance.

Occupational therapy

Throughout the whole of the rehabilitation period the OT is working to improve muscle strength in the lower and upper limbs, to improve stamina and endurance and to improve balance and co-ordination of movement. Activities of daily living (ADL) are practised in the ward and department and clothes may need to be adapted at this time.

Bed. In the ward the OT will ensure that bed equipment aids are available for the patient's use. These may include monkey poles, rope ladders and possibly cot sides for the bilateral amputee. These equipment aids will be attached to a low, firm bed which will assist the patient to transfer and move about in the bed.

Personal. The OT will also work with nursing staff to ensure that the patient attends to his personal care (e.g. washing, shaving and dressing) as soon as possible. Again, equipment aids may have to be supplied and advice given on how to dress safely. Patients are encouraged to dress the top halves of their bodies initially in the early post-operative days and progress to pants and trousers or skirts, which are more difficult, especially for the bilateral amputee (Conder, 1987).

Wheelchairs. Wheelchairs are loaned pre-operatively or in the first day or two to patients who do not have one of their own. This helps the patients to strengthen their upper limbs and enables them to become independently mobile and widen their hospital environment and therefore interest. It is advisable for every occupational therapy department in the UK to have a wheelchair store of loan chairs, as standard models take 31 days on average to be delivered (Ham, 1987). On issuing the wheelchair, the patient should be taught the following: how to apply and release the brakes, rotate and remove the foot rests and arm rests for transfers, transfer from the bed to chair and chair to toilet safely, propel the wheelchair through doorways, narrow spaces and turn in the chair. It is also advisable to teach the patient or a relative at some time during their hospital stay, how to fold and lift the chair for transportation and storage. Wheelchair training and provision is carried out by either therapist and not specifically the OT.

The centre of gravity of bilateral amputees have moved backwards as they have lost the weight of their legs. To prevent these patients tipping backwards in the wheelchair they should be provided with a model that has the rear wheels set back by three inches. This type of wheelchair may also be required for a tall patient to prevent them tipping backwards when they propel. It may also be necessary to loan a bilateral amputee a wheelchair seat belt for general use in the hospital or for outings with his family or for weekend leave. All patients should be loaned a cushion for the wheelchair. In the UK, this may be the standard government two inch cushion or it may be a more sophisticated one, necessary for pressure relief and the prevention of pressure sores, for the bilateral for example. The majority of amputees will require a wheelchair for the future even if they are to become prosthetic users, to maintain their mobility. In the UK, wheelchairs are available from the state and are now obtained locally.

Transfers. The OT will teach the patient to transfer from bed to wheelchair, wheelchair to toilet and wheelchair to bath. These will be practised in the ward and therapy departments to increase the patient's confidence and subsequent independence. The OT liaises with the PT so that activities are not duplicated unless their repetition is necessary for functional independence. The bilateral amputee will require more practice and also therefore more time (Conder, 1987).

Psychological support. The OT should be aware of the adjustment and bereavement process through which the amputee is going, as their psychological state will influence their level of independence and motivation to progress. Support may take the form of informal counselling with the patient or their family or it may involve more practical action, for example giving the patient the opportunity to do his own washing or bake something for the family (Chapter 10).

Therapeutic activity. Activities such as woodwork, cooking, printing or remedial games are used at this stage to help to improve the patient's physical function which in turn will enable the patient to achieve maximum independence in his daily living skills.

It is important that all staff hide any revulsion that they may feel at the sight of the open stump. Touching the stump by the staff and the patient will help the patient overcome any similar feelings he may have initially. Whenever possible appointment times for therapy can be given to the patient to increase his independence.

Early home visit

In the first post-operative week the PT, OT or social worker will visit the patient's home without the patient but with his permission and knowledge. The purpose of this visit is to assess the patient's accommodation, noting the possibility and equipment requirements for weekend leave and recording the necessary adaptations and aids that will be necessary before discharge is possible. If rehousing or a housing transfer are necessary this can be brought to the attention of the rest of the team, but especially the social worker.

This early home visit has also been found to be a very useful time to meet and talk to the patient's family and friends outside the alien hospital environment and to learn more about the patient, his possible attitude to disability and the problems or family concerns that may arise when he is ready for discharge. A report of the early home visit is given to all team members at the weekly meeting and copies are generally kept in the patient's medical and therapeutic notes.

Weekly meeting

For a team approach to work well weekly meetings are essential. Brief details of the patients undergoing treatment may be circulated at the meeting for discussion and short- and long-term goals can be reassessed and noted. In a teaching hospital these weekly team meetings should also be used as a teaching forum and students should be encouraged to attend.

Early walking aids

The prolonged immobilization of patients in hospital, especially the elderly, prior to rehabilitation is detrimental to successful rehabilitation, therefore it is imperative that patients should be mobilized as soon as possible (Acton *et al.*, 1984). Elderly patients also have problems of the cardiovascular and locomotor systems which prevent them from hopping functionally on one leg. Hopping on this remaining leg is also undesirable since its circulation is usually also impaired (Dickstein *et al.*, 1982). It is therefore important when rehabilitating an amputee that mobilization takes place on two limbs using a bipedal gait. Early walking aids have been developed over the last 10 years as tools to provide this function and to relieve pressure on the remaining limb (Dickstein *et al.*, 1982). Their purpose is three-fold. They help to assess the patient's ability, physical capability and motivation for using a prosthesis. They are useful pieces of equipment to provide the first possibilities of exercising the patient in standing and walking with a bipedal gait. Both of these activities help the patient a great deal psychologically in his rehabilitation programme. With regular use, early walking aids also help reduce stump oedema and the associated stump pain.

There are four types of early walking aid available.

1. The first type is pneumatic, using air bags. Examples of these are the Vessa Ppam Aid, the Jobst Air Splint and the Airleg.
2. The second type are in total contact using a vacuum technique, for example the LIC Tulip for the below-knee amputee.
3. The third type uses preformed laminated plastic sockets, the LIC Femurett for example, for the above-knee amputee.
4. Local varieties.

1. Pneumatic devices.
The Vessa Ppam Aid (Vessa Ltd., Paper Mill Lane, Alton, Hampshire GU34 2PY, UK)
The Ppam Aid equipment consists of a small cushion inner bag and larger above- and below-knee bags (Figure 8.2). The bags are encased in an outer metal frame which comes in three sizes: short, medium and long. The frames have a crucible sling support on their distal end and a shoulder support strap. The equipment set is completed with a foot pump with a dial measuring pressure in mmHg.

The stump is assessed by the surgeon and the PT and once stable and healing without complications, approximately 5–10 days post-operatively, the use of the Ppam Aid begins. Nursing staff are informed and daily inspection of the wound by the nurses and PT is carried out to ensure that the healing rate continues.

On the first application, the appropriate length bag with the small cushion bag and metal frame are applied, with the patient commonly in

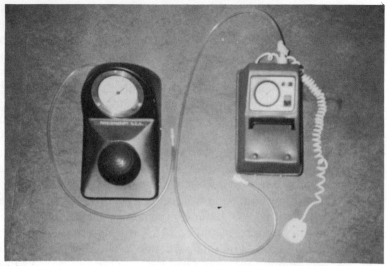

(a)

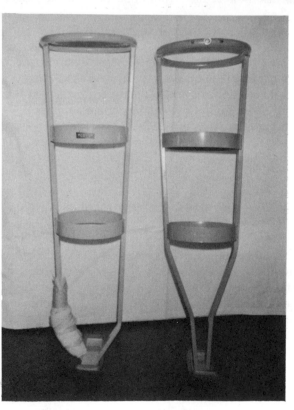

(b)

Figure 8.2 The original and modified Vessa Ppam Aid. (a) Left, original; right, modified, (b) left, original; right, modified.

a half lying position on a plinth. The pressure is slowly increased to the maximum the patient can tolerate. On the first application this is usually between 15 and 25 mmHg for approximately 5 and 10 minutes. If the amount of discomfort the patient feels increases, the bag is deflated and reapplied. The patient's attitude to amputation, recovery, disability and the amount of discomfort he is experiencing all play a part in the speed of his rehabilitation.

If there are no ischaemic areas, the wound is healing well and the amount of discharge is acceptable, the length of time the Ppam Aid is used is increased. When the patient can tolerate 40 mmHg then standing balance exercises using a mirror and walking between parallel bars can begin.

Between the seventh and fourteenth day the amount of time the patient uses the device increases but only in conjunction with his routine mobilizing and strengthening exercises and not instead of these. If the wound is oozing a little, its use will continue. Daily inspection of stumps ensures that therapy is helping to promote healing rather than causing the stump to break down. Emphasis on the following points should be made during gait training: leading with the unaffected leg, an even step length, hip hitching (lifting the leg from the pelvis, keeping the knee extended) and an upright posture. As the device is designed as a partial weight-bearing aid and as the bags have been known to burst it is recommended that the younger, fitter patients use the device out of the parallel bars using elbow crutches. Good balance reactions for this are essential.

When used carefully the Ppam Aid is a very useful tool. When used incorrectly on stumps that are not mature enough and for far too long a period, the device can be dangerous, often leading to delayed healing or even reamputation at a higher level. Caution is therefore required with its application and regular monitoring and inspection of the stump is essential.

Objectively, it appears that oedema is reduced, wound healing is not impaired and volume change in the stump is reduced, permitting a definitive socket to be made at an earlier stage (Redhead, 1983). Modifications to the equipment have been made since its original design (Ham *et al.*, 1989).

The Jobst Air Splint (Jobst Institute Inc., 653 Miami St., Toledo, OH 43605, USA)
The Jobst Air Splint equipment consists of a clear plastic tube with a zipper front that is tapered and sealed at the base. The splint is inflated by a foot pump with a manometer in series.

The Air Splint can be applied at surgery but is often not applied until between 2 and 10 days post-operatively. Pressures can be maintained at rest between 25 and 30 mmHg and increased to 50 mmHg for ambulation (Rausch and Khalili, 1985). Other centres apply the splint initially for 3 hours twice a day, gradually increasing to all day, removing it for 3 hours only. Its advantages are that equal pressure is maintained, it is self-suspending, light and easy to apply, allows for early ambulation and helps to prevent flexion contractures for the below-knee amputee. It is, however, cumbersome, hot to wear, difficult to suspend for the above-knee amputee, difficult to turn in bed and the bags are prone to leakage.

The Airleg (M.K. Henderson Industries Inc., PO Box 245, Radnor PA 19087, USA)

The Airleg was developed by Francis J. Bonner Sr and his associates. It consists of two parts: an inner air sac and a quadrilateral outer shell of fibreglass with a metal shank and prosthetic foot. The air sac is applied immediately following amputation over a soft dressing and pressure maintained at 12 mmHg. It is worn 24 hours a day and removed only for wound inspection and dressing changes. The outer temporary prosthesis is applied for ambulation and the pressure is increased to 25–30 mmHg. The advantages of the Airleg is that it is light and may be applied by staff with minimal training. It provides constant measurable pressure and total contact, reducing stump trauma. The Airleg acts as a shock absorber, allowing weight bearing of greater than 9 kg. The quadrilateral design of the fibreglass external shell with its attached prosthetic foot, provides improved stability and increases weight bearing. It is possible to treat open or ulcerated stumps with the Airleg (Bonner and Green, 1982).

The systems disadvantages are that air leakage occurs after a period of time and excessive perspiration can be a problem, especially in hot weather.

2. Vacuum devices.

LIC Tulip limb (LIC Orthopaedic, S-171 83 Solna, Sweden)

The LIC Tulip limb (Figure 8.3) for the below-knee amputee was developed in Sweden in 1978 (Henriksen et al., 1978). The equipment is composed of an inner cushion bag in four sections which contain small plastic pellets, a rigid adjustable four petal or 'tulip' frame made from polypropylene, with an adjustable tube and a single axis foot and a pump. The inner bag is wrapped around the dressed stump, evacuated of air by the pump and then wrapped with a bandage. The tulip socket is

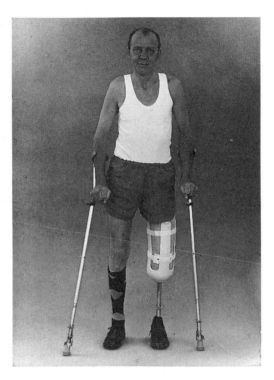

Figure 8.3 LIC Tulip limb.

then applied, 10–20 cm above the knee joint line and the tube is adjusted to the correct length with the velcro bands applied to control the width and patella tendon support.

The Tulip serves as a semi rigid support and it is used for 30–60 minutes at a time, 2–3 weeks post-operatively (Leidberg *et al.*, 1983). As with other early walking aids, it is used until a definitive prosthesis is delivered to the patient.

3. Preformed sockets.

The LIC Femorett (LIC Orthopaedic, S-171 83 Solna, Sweden)

The Femorett (Figure 8.4) consists of a neutral uniaxial ankle and foot, a tubular lower leg section adjustable for length and foot rotation, a single axis knee joint with extension spring and lock, a thigh section

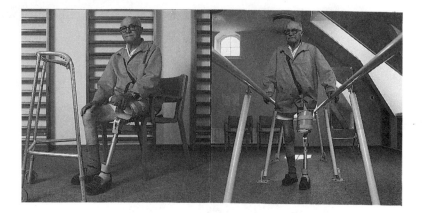

Figure 8.4 LIC Femurett.

adjustable for length and rotation, three different sizes of adjustable quadrilateral socket for left or right fittings and a shoulder strap.

The advantages of the system are that it is light, relatively easy to apply with minimal training and the hard socket with the ischial seat provides greater rigidity and security to the patient than, for example, the Ppam Aid (Parry and Morrison, 1989).

The foot is of psychological benefit and its use reduces the days it takes for the patient to reach independence. Its disadvantages are that it costs the same as a definitive above-knee prosthesis, the knee extension spring mechanism is too strong to allow walking with a free knee and it does not control oedema as well as the Vessa Ppam Aid. As with other early walking aids it can be used as an assessment tool and for walking training prior to receiving the definitive prosthesis.

4. Local varieties. Other walking aids have been produced in areas where, for example, limb fitting contact was at a distance. These include The London Hospital early walking aid, consisting of a stump corset made of Johnson and Johnson's Orthoplast which is directly moulded onto the individual to form an ischial shelf. Two duraluminium struts measured to the required length are attached to the corset and a wooden rocker used as a foot piece (Acton *et al.*, 1984). Its length and circumference are variable during rehabilitation.

In the Reading area of England, an early walking device was developed to overcome transportation problems (Hutton and Rothnie, 1977). This device consists of a socket of either padded leather or metal to which is attached a body belt and side irons leading to a lockable knee joint. The side irons are fixed at the lower end to a semi-flexible foot piece or a simple rocker.

A similar device was developed in Hastings consisting of a polyethylene socket, two side steels leading to joints, a reclaimed calf piece from a prosthesis and a foot or simple rocker (Devas, 1971). The socket is usually lined with plastic foam and a waist belt is fixed to the top of the socket with a swivel joint.

The LIC LEMA (Figure 8.5) prosthesis is a similar device, though more modern, which is made from a polypropylene socket, side steels (with or without a hinged knee joint) and a foot.

A Hexelite temporary patella tendon-bearing (PTB) prosthesis has also been developed. The Hexelite is immersed in hot water then wrapped around the stump in the same way as a PTB socket is wrap cast. It is then left to cool and harden and a shank, foot and suspension

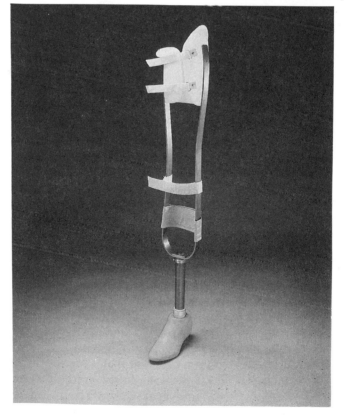

Figure 8.5 LIC LEMA.

strap are riveted onto the socket and the prosthesis is ready for use (Callen, 1981). A similar below-knee device, the Halmstad prosthesis, is available through LIC (Ham, 1988).

Lightcast II, an orthopaedic casting system consisting of an open weave fibreglass tape impregnated with a photosensitive resin which hardens in 3 minutes when exposed to light has also been used to make temporary lower limb prostheses (Ruder *et al.*, 1977). The socket, once cast, has an Otto Bock modular endoskeletal prosthetic system attached to it for use. The material is strong, porous and fairly easy to use. Scotcast and polyvinyl and chloride interim prostheses for below-knee amputees have also been reported (Wu *et al.*, 1981).

The early walking aid that is chosen to exercise, assess and speed up the patient's rehabilitation is dependent on local circumstances and the personal preference of the PT and surgeon. It is used in the first few weeks of the rehabilitation process in conjunction with an exercise strengthening and mobilizing programme. Until the stump is healed and sutures removed, weight bearing should be restricted.

Group therapy

The value of group support for patients with disabling or chronic illness has been known for a long time. Meeting others teaches patients about their diseases and allows them to express feelings about their shared experiences. Meetings help to assist with feelings of isolation, helplessness and depression and facilitate staff awareness of psychological factors in each patient's rehabilitation. The meetings integrate ward and therapy treatments and help to mobilize the patient's coping skills. They also help the patient to participate in the rehabilitation of other amputees. One example may be the recall meeting. The therapists may work with the social worker to arrange amputee group meetings where a specific topic may be discussed or an invited speaker leads the meeting. In- and out-patients may attend and it gives new amputees an opportunity to ask experienced amputees and their families specific questions. Often it is simply reassurance that is needed and greater notice is taken of advice from a fellow amputee than from staff. Patients have said repeatedly that weekly group meetings involving both new and established amputees, are more pertinent and helpful than the encouragement they received from staff and their families (MacBride *et al.*, 1980). Tea and coffee at such sessions has been found to help relax the atmosphere, and 8–12 amputees and one to three members of staff has been found to be a good number for such meetings (Lipp and Malone, 1976).

Late post-operative period

The patient's exercise programme is extended as his condition improves and this should be regularly reviewed and, whenever possible, the patient should take an active part in his own progress. It is important that the following groups of muscles are exercised.

1. The hip extensors are necessary to hold the knee stable in the stance phase. This may be practised when side lying or prone lying, at first actively with verbal encouragement and then actively with resistance. This may be using springs in which case the patient may be positioned in long sitting on a plinth or using balls lying supine on a plinth. Modified proprioceptive neuromuscular facilitation (PNF) patterns may also be used.

2. The hip flexors are necessary to accelerate the leg forward, to initiate control of an articulated knee joint, for stair walking and for sitting to standing. Above-knee amputees, especially, tend to hold their stumps flexed at the hip. This should be discouraged but active exercises to strengthen the hip flexors and increase the range of hip movement should be actively practised in association with hip extension.

3. The hip abductors and adductors are necessary for stability in stance. Both of these groups may be strengthened by actively resisting the movement with PNF patterns or by using equipment such as sandbags or balls in the appropriate starting position.

4. The knee flexors are necessary for knee stabilization on weight bearing and to decelerate the leg's forward motion before heel contact. Below-knee amputees tend to hold their stumps in flexion. This should be avoided and active flexion/extension exercises should be practised. This may be in the supine position using a soft ball or using manual resistance, perhaps with PNF.

5. The hip extensors are necessary for heel contact at heel strike and for stability in stance. Initially this movement may be practised actively over a pillow or block then actively with resistance, perhaps using springs, manual resistance or PNF. For the more active patient a multigym system may be appropriate. All the exercises should be progressed and the patient should be aware of his progress and the importance of the exercises. Individual weakness should be highlighted with the patient so that a personal programme can be followed. Details

121

of specific exercises are not given here as good descriptions are given elsewhere (Engstrom and Van de Ven, 1985).

For the elderly patients, a basic programme will be less confusing and provide them with exercises they can perform on the ward alone and at weekends. For the younger patient a more active and variable programme will be appropriate. For all patients a record of exercise progression and therefore increasing physical capability that they can understand will help to motivate them during this period of rehabilitation. Younger patients may find sport and recreation rewarding, particularly swimming. Also during this period, weekend leave or day leave is recommended as it breaks the monotomy of hospital life and helps the amputee and his family become accustomed to the new situation (Hutton and Rothnie, 1977).

Prosthetic referral

It is recommended that the PT records the stump volume measurements of patients who are suitable for a prosthesis at least twice a week to check that the volume is reducing. This can be done crudely with a tape measure, marking an anatomical landmark, for example the superior border of the patella, and then taking circumferential measurements at set intervals below this landmark on the stump. When the stump volume is stable and the wound satisfactory the patient is ready to be measured for a prosthesis.

For the patients who are personally independent (i.e. who dress, wash and toilet, show motivation and an ability to use an early walking aid), a referral for prosthetic prescription is made. In the UK this is done in a variety of ways, using a government AOF3 form which is sent to the prosthetic centre, or through a satellite clinic or visiting service where referral is on a verbal basis.

The bilateral amputee – the non-walker

As the majority of amputations in the west are for vascular disease in the elderly population, it is now increasingly common to see amputees who have lost both legs. In a number of recently published studies the time from losing the first limb to losing the second varied from 6 months (Ebskov, 1986) to 5 years (Dormandy and Thomas, 1988). The percentages of patients losing their second leg also varies from 10% in 1 year (Sanders, 1986) to 77% in 2 years (Boontje, 1980).

For the bilateral amputee it is essential that the therapist teaches the

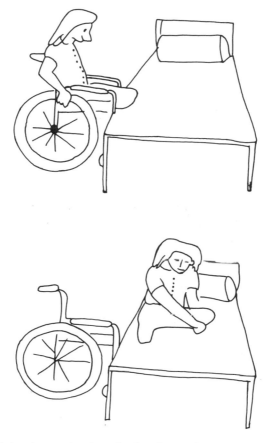

Figure 8.6 Bilateral amputee transferring forwards.

patient rolling and bed mobility, arm exercises, balance re-education, transfers and wheelchair manoeuvres in the early rehabilitation phase. For ease and safety the majority of bilaterals transfer forwards onto the bed and toilet and backwards onto the wheelchair (Figure 8.6). Their comfort in the wheelchair must be assessed and their safety in the chair and during transportation must be checked. During the home visit the height of surfaces for transfers and functional activities must be considered as well as access and community support. Electric wheelchairs should be considered for this group of patients if this will increase their quality of life. As their mobility has decreased, a range of appropriate chairbound activities will be introduced to them by the OT.

All amputees consume more oxygen walking than the normal subject and this is greatest for the bilateral amputee. Propelling a wheelchair consumes less oxygen than walking. It is therefore essential that the bilateral amputee has a careful and thorough assessment before prescribing prostheses. 'There is little point in supplying prostheses or even teaching a patient to use prostheses if he will never be able to put them on without help' (Van de Ven, 1981).

In a series of 103 vascular patients, the author reported that of 35 bilateral above-knee amputees, 22 remained in wheelchairs and 13 were bedridden. Of the 21 bilateral above- and below-knee amputees, 5 became prosthetic users, 10 wheelchair cases and 6 remained bedridden. Of the remaining 44 bilateral below-knee amputees, 35 became prosthetic users and 9 were wheelchair bound (Volpicelli *et al.*, 1983). Preservation of the knee joint is therefore very important as walking without at least one knee joint is almost impossible. Rehabilitation of the bilateral amputee also takes longer. For example, in a series of 44 patients, 65% became totally independent, but their mean rehabilitation time was 30 weeks (26–78 weeks) (Kerstein *et al.*, 1975).

THE PROSTHETIC TRAINING PHASE

In the UK it has been estimated that there are almost 10 000 new amputees per annum (Dormandy and Thomas, 1988). Of these, almost 5500 attend Prosthetic Centres for prosthetic prescription. Ninety-four per cent of those sent to the centres are fitted with prostheses (Day, 1982). The remaining 6% are technically or medically impossible to fit, medically unsuitable or do not want a leg. It is essential that only patients who are 'able' to use a prosthesis are prescribed one. A good team approach will ensure that only the patients who can manage a prosthesis will be prescribed one.

Gait training

Once the patient receives his prosthesis meticulous attention to detail during the training programme is necessary (Steinberg *et al.*, 1985). Training periods should be daily and not two or three times a week, and run for a whole day with a lunch-time break period. The training should include periods of walking and rest and the stump should be inspected several times a day for signs of irritation that may require attention (Sanders, 1986). For the elderly amputee especially, methods of reinforcement of training procedures are helpful, for example written and pictorial as well as verbal (Edelstein, 1987). Including the family in at least some of these sessions will help ensure that prosthetic use continues following discharge.

The amputee is shown the variety of socks that are available, cotton, towelling, wool and nylon, and taught how to interchange them with the shrinkage and swelling in the stump. He is taught how to put on and take off his prosthesis, initially in the physiotherapy gym and then in the ward. Balance re-education, weight transference onto the prosthesis and walking are taught initially in the parallel bars with a mirror. Once the patient is stable and walking well in parallel bars, he starts to walk in the gym with a suitable walking aid. It is important that from an early stage, amputees are taught to bear weight correctly through their prosthesis. Three point gait, generally used for partial weight bearing should therefore be avoided. Specific exercises for each prosthetic level are given in Chapter 12.

Gait training is continued to include a variety of surfaces and then practised outdoors. Stairs and slopes are taught at the appropriate time and all patients should be taught how to get up from the floor in case of a fall.

FUNCTIONAL ACTIVITIES

Activities of daily living

Once the patient has received his prosthesis, activities of daily living should be reassessed to ensure continued independence. The patient may need further instruction in dressing with the prosthesis and clothing may need to be altered. Often the male patients require braces to assist them with fastening their trousers and balancing simultaneously.

Kitchen

In the kitchen the activities practised range from making a drink to cooking a lunch. For the single amputee who walks, few alterations to the kitchen are needed. A perching stool and a trolley are useful to the single amputee who is a poor prosthetic user. The bilateral amputee may need many alterations to their home, for example work surfaces lowered to wheelchair height, an alternative cooker that can be managed from a chair and tap and window extension levers. Plugs and shelves may also have to be altered for access from a wheelchair.

Although activities are practised in the hospital setting it is essential that they are also related to the patient's home environment. This is made easier for the therapist when she has seen the home at an early home visit.

Therapeutic activity

Once the patient has a prosthesis such activities are planned to improve the patient's standing balance and tolerance (Leason, 1989, personal communication).

HOME VISIT

When the patient is almost fully independent, either on a prosthesis or from a wheelchair, a home visit is arranged, generally between the OT and PT. This is to ensure that all activities of daily living are checked at home as well as access, accommodation, equipment and the social services support requirements. Once the patient is fully independent and all requests delivered, a discharge date approximately one week in advance is made to finalize the discharge plans and allow the family time to prepare. A report from the visit is prepared and circulated to the relevant members of the team. Prior to discharge it is essential for the general practitioner and community staff to receive a discharge summary (Appendix 8.2) so that they are aware of the rehabilitation and future plans for that individual patient. Each patient requires a hospital contact and this is often the PT due to the long-standing relationship that has developed (Condie, 1988).

The most typical aids required for amputees are toilet-seat raise, non-slip bath mat, bath board and seat, commode, grab-rails by the toilet, a step or stair rails, bed blocks, social service-type easy chair, outdoor wheelchair ramps, glideabout chairs, helping hand, and kitchen trolley. Double amputees often require two bath boards but no seat, with a shower attachment, a fixed scandia around the toilet, raised electric sockets, lowered light switches, outdoor wheelchair ramps with rails, a bed rope ladder, monkey pole, wheelchair cushions, wheelchair seat belts, double sliding boards for car access, alteration in work-top heights and storage space, and adaptation to clothes, especially underpants.

Aids and adaptations are requested through the community OT and the completion of the work requested is often checked by her. When patients are from well outside the catchment area it is generally the local OT who is contacted by the hospital staff and asked to visit the house and assess for suitable aids. She will provide these prior to discharge or visit the patient following discharge.

It is important to remember that discharge is usually a stressful point in rehabilitation. The patients should be reassured that they will not be discharged without sound pre-planning. It is also beneficial to involve the patients in some of the decision making for their discharge, to allow them to take some responsibility.

A study in 1978 in the USA reviewed 134 patients 6 months to 12 years following their amputation, to assess their activities of daily living. Three per cent needed help dressing, 55% help with bathing, 56% help with transfers and 60% required chairs with arms to assist transfers. Eighty-seven per cent of the patients had not changed their original accommodation. The length of time from amputation had no additional effect in determining the functional outcome and the authors recommended that more bathing practice, home visits, group discussions with staff and a written list of local resources should be offered prior to discharge (Kegel *et al.*, 1978). In a recent study in the UK of below-knee patients, 47% of the amputees discharged required no alterations to their homes, 32% required some alterations and 13% were re-housed (de Cossart *et al.*, 1983).

OTHER CONSIDERATIONS

Disablement resettlement officer

If the patient is returning to work, the disablement resettlement officer (DRO) may be contacted to help resolve any problems with the employer regarding the disability or problems on the work site. The DRO will generally liaise with the OT and social worker (Leason, 1989, personal communication).

Driving

The patient may need to be put in touch with a specialist centre to advise them on car adaptations. The amputee's needs will vary depending upon the site of amputation. Car insurance companies will also need to be contacted (Ham and Kerfoot, 1989).

OUT-PATIENT PHYSIOTHERAPY

Whenever possible, amputees should remain in hospital until they are fully independent from a wheelchair or using a prosthesis. On discharge they should only need to return for physiotherapy when they receive a more sophisticated prosthesis or require a few extra sessions to gain their confidence following a setback, for example a fall. If patients are discharged before becoming fully independent, daily out-patient sessions should be planned for a short period; not twice a week for months due to inevitable staff changes. Goals should be set that are realistic. The patient and his family must be kept informed and involved with plans as they are discussed and made.

Follow-up visit

Following discharge a follow-up visit is often needed to check on any new practical problems, such as the equipment location and any new anxiety or feelings that may have arisen. This is often done by the OT at 1–2 weeks following discharge. Periodical reviews are necessary of all the patients to ensure that they are not having problems and patients should be regarded as the hospital department's patients 'until death do us part' (Hunter, 1986, personal communication).

The outcome of rehabilitation is a multifaceted phenomenon comprising medical, social, vocational and psychological aspects (Gerhards *et al.*, 1984). Risk factors that may increase the problems of unsatisfactory rehabilitation may be as follows:

1. poor social integration;
2. introverted and withdrawn personality;
3. little athletic activity;
4. low level risk taking;
5. 'amputation' being thought the fault of others and no insight into its necessity;
6. unstable partnership;
7. no person to confide in;
8. a non-specialist hospital;
9. several reamputations; and
10. time lapses between amputation and prosthetic fitting.

There is a direct relationship between achievement and co-operation. Disabled people work hardest for recovery when there is a home and someone who loves them waiting. If there is no-one to perform for and nowhere to go, patients become dependent and passive. Emotional factors and a degree of acceptance of amputation will determine the training rate and potential achievement (Russek, 1961).

REFERENCES

Acton, D., Hyland, J., Nolan, D. and Bouchier-Hayes, D. (1984) In-hospital rehabilitation of amputees: a prospective study. *Irish Med. J.*, **77**, 131–133.

Atkinson, H.W. (1974) Assessing the patient, in *Neurology for Physiotherapists* (ed. J. Cash), Faber, London, 85 pp.

Browse, N.L. (1974) Amputation of the lower limb. *Nursing Mirror*, 7 June, 63–65.

Bonner, F.T. Jr and Green, R.F. (1982) Pneumatic airleg prosthesis: report of 200 cases. *Arch. Phys. Med. Rehabil.*, **63**, 383–385.

Boontje, A.A. (1980) Major amputations of the lower extremity for vascular disease. *Prosthet. Orthot. Int.*, **4**, 87–89.

Burgess, E.M. and Alexander, A.G. (1973) The expanding role of the physical therapist on the amputee rehabilitation team. *Phys. Ther.*, **53**, 141–143.

Callen, S. (1981) Hexcelite temporary prosthesis for lower-limb amputees. *Physiotherapy*, **67**, 138–139.

Chi-Tsou, H., Jackson, J.R., Moore, N.B., Fine, P.R., Kuhlemeier, K.V., Traugh, G.H. and Saunders, P.T. (1979) Amputation energy cost of ambulation. *Arch. Phys. Med. Rehabil.*, **60**, 18–24.

Conder, D. (1987) Amputation. Lower and upper limb, in *Practice of Occupational Therapy* (ed. A. Turner), Churchill Livingstone, Edinburgh, pp. 271–294.

Condie, E. (1988) Physiotherapy and the lower limb amputee, in *Amputation Surgery and Lower Limb Prosthetics* (ed. G. Murdoch), Blackwell Scientific, Oxford, pp. 71–80.

Day, H.J.B. (1982) Rehabilitation of the elderly amputee. *Geriatric Medicine*, May 1982, 26–31.

de Cossart, L., Randall, P., Turner, P. and Marcuson, R.W. (1983) The fate of the below knee amputee. *Ann. R. Coll. Surg. (Eng.)*, **65**, 230–232.

Devas, M.B. (1971) Early walking of geriatric amputees. *Br. Med. J.*, **1**, 394–396.

Dickstein, R., Pillar, T. and Mannheim, M. (1982) The pneumatic postamputation aid in geriatric rehabilitation. *Scand. J. Rehab. Med.*, **14**, 149–150.

Dormandy, J.A. and Thomas, P.R.S. (1988) What is the natural history of a critically ischaemic patient with and without his leg?, in *Limb Salvage and Amputation for Vascular Disease* (eds R.M. Greenhalgh, C.W. Jamieson and A.N. Nicholaides), Saunders, London, pp. 11–28.

Ebskov, B. (1986) The Danish amputation register 1972–1984. *Prosthet. Orthot. Int.*, **10**, 40–42.

Edelstein, J.E. (1987) Realistic management of the older amputee. *Top. Geriatr. Rehabil.*, **2**, 29–44.

Engstrom, B. and Van de Ven, C. (1985) Exercise programmes in the department, in *Physiotherapy for Amputees. The Roehampton Approach.* Churchill Livingstone, Edinburgh, pp. 37–55.

Gerhards, F., Florin, I. and Knapp, T. (1984) The impact of medical, re-educational and psychological variables on rehabilitation outcomes in amputees. *Int. J. Rehab. Res.*, **7**, 379–388.

Ham, R. (1987) Wheelchair provision in a London health authority. *Physiotherapy*, **73**, 576–578.

Ham, R.O. (1988) Amputee rehabilitation: a review of practice in Denmark and Sweden, in *Council of Europe Medical Fellowship*, No. 88062, pp. 28–29, 32.

Ham, R. and Richardson, P. (1986) The King's amputee stump board—Mark II. *Physiotherapy*, **72**, 124.

Ham, R. and Kerfoot, S. (1989) *Recovering from Amputation – the Dulwich Way*, Kings College School of Medicine and Dentistry, London SE5.

Ham, R., Richardson, P. and Sweet, A. (1989) A new look at the Vessa Ppam Aid. *Physiotherapy*, **75**, 493–494.

Hamilton, A. (1977) Device for supporting the stump of a below-knee amputee. *Physiotherapy*, **63**, 320.

Henriksen, O., Marsch, G. and Persson, B. (1978) The Tulip prosthesis. *Acta Orthop. Scand.*, **47**, 107.

Hutton, I.M. and Rothnie, N.G. (1977) The early mobilisation in the elderly amputee, *Br. J. Surg.*, **64**, 267–270.

Kegel, B., Carpenter, M.L. and Burgess, E.M. (1978) Functional capabilities of lower extremity amputees. *Arch. Phys. Med. Rehabil.*, **59**, 109–120.

Kerstein, M.D., Zimmer, H., Dugdale, F.E. and Lerner, E. (1975) Rehabilitation after bilateral lower-extremity amputation. *Arch. Phys. Med. Rehabil.*, **56**, 309–311.

Leidberg, E., Hommerberg, H. and Persson, B.M. (1983) The tolerance of early walking and total contact among below-knee amputees – a randomised test. *Prosthet. Orthot. Int.*, **7**, 91–95.

Lipp, M.R. and Malone, S.T. (1976) Group rehabilitation of vascular surgery patients. *Arch. Phys. Med. Rehabil.*, **57**, 180–183.

MacBride, A., Rogers, J., Whylie, B. and Freenman, S.J.J. (1980) Psychological factors in the rehabilitation of elderly amputees. *Psychosomatics*, **21**, 258–265.

Mensch, G. and Ellis, P.M. (1987) Preoperative and postoperative care and the responsibility of the physical therapist, in *Physical Therapy Management of Lower Extremity Amputations.* Heinemann Physiotherapy, London, pp. 45–200.

Parry, M. and Morrison, J.D. (1989) Use of the Femurett adjustable prosthesis in the assessment and walking training of new above-knee amputees. *Prosthet. Orthot. Int.*, **13**, 36–38.

Rausch, R.W. and Khalili, A.A. (1985) Air splint in preprosthetic rehabilitation of lower extremity amputated limbs. *Phys. Ther.*, **65**, 912–914.

Redhead, R.G. (1983) The early rehabilitation of lower limb amputees using a pneumatic walking aid. *Prosthet. Orthot. Int.*, **7**, 88–90.

Ruder, K., Fernie, G.R. and Kostuik, J.P. (1977) Techniques of lower limb prosthetic manufacture using highcast II. *Prosthet. Orthot. Int.*, **1**, 84–88.

Russek, A.S. (1961) Management of lower extremity amputees. *Arch. Phys. Med. Rehabil.*, 687–703.

Steinberg, F.U., Sunwoo, I. and Roettger, R.F. (1985) Prosthetic rehabilitation of geriatric amputee patients: a follow-up study. *Arch. Phys. Med. Rehabil.*, **66**, 742–745.

Troop, I.M. and Wood, M.A. (1982) Physiotherapy, in *Total Care of the Lower Limb Amputee*, Pitman Books, London, pp. 104–117.

Volpicelli, L.J., Chambers, R.B. and Wagner, F.W. (1983) Ambulation levels of bilateral lower-extremity amputees. *J. Bone Joint Surg.*, **65**, 599–605.

Wu, Y., Binack, M.D., Krick, H.J, Pitman, T.D. and Stratigos, J.S. (1981) Scotchcast PVC interim prosthesis for below-knee amputees. *Bull. Prosthet. Res.*, fall 1981, 10–36, 40–45.

APPENDIX 8.1: AMPUTEE ASSESSMENT

Name: . . . .   Consultant: . . . .

Address: . . . .   Hospital No: . . . .

. . . .   L.F.C. No: . . . .

. . . .   D.O.B.: . . . .

Tel. No: . . . .   Last occupation: . . . .

Date of admission: . . . .

GP: . . . .   Amputation date: . . . .

Address: . . . .

. . . .

. . . .

Tel. No: . . . .

Contact telephone numbers, i.e. friends/family

Social Services   Area No: Tel. No:
   Area OT
   Area SW
   District Nurse

Present Social Services
   Home help
   Meals on wheels
   Day centre
   Luncheon club

Accommodation

House	Own
Part of a house	Rented
Bungalow	Council
Flat	With spouse
Sheltered	With family
Part III	Alone
Hostel	

Amenities
Bathroom
  Access
Toilet
  Access

Stairs/steps
Indoor
Outdoor
Lift

Pre-admission independence
Dressing
Toilet
Bath
Stairs
Shopping
Cooking

Mobility
Last walked – Indoor and distance
         – Outdoor and distance
Aids for walking
Wheelchair

Aids currently provided
Toilet
Bath
Bedroom
Sitting room
Kitchen

Medical history
Diagnosis:

Previous medical history

Present admission

Amputation date:
Anaesthetic:
Smoking habit:
Sight:
Hearing:
Mental state:

Legs	*Affected*		*Unaffected*
		Hip joint	
		Knee joint	
		Ankle joint	
		Skin	
		Sensation	
		Pressure areas	

Arms	*Left*		*Right*
		Shoulder joint	
		Elbow joint	
		Wrist joint	
		Hand/grip	
		Skin/sensation	

Artificial limb
Type:

Date assessed and measured:

Date received:

At discharge
  Dress
  Toilet
  Bath
  Put limb on (don)

Take limb off (doff)
Stairs
Slopes
Rough ground
Get up off floor
Wheelchair control
Hop with crutches (if appropriate)
Mobility at discharge

Date of early home visit:
Date of home visit:
Date of discharge:
Out-patient physiotherapy:
Date discharge summary sent to GP:
Aids necessary for discharge:

Social Services arranged for discharge:

APPENDIX 8.2: COMMUNITY DISCHARGE SUMMARY

Name: . . . .   D.O.B.: . . . .

Address: . . . .   Consultant: . . . .

. . . .   Ward: . . . .

. . . .   Date of admission: . . . .

Diagnosis: . . . .

Date of amputation: . . . .

Tel: . . . .   Date of discharge: . . . .

GP: . . . .

Address: . . . .

. . . .

. . . .

Discharge arrangements for the above-named patient have been made as follows:

District Nurse:

Social Services   Area No: Tel. No:
    Social Worker involved:
    Referred for the following:
        Home help
        Meals on wheels
        Day centre
        Luncheon club
        Other

Housing
    As before
    Sheltered accommodation
    Housing transfer
    Residential home (Part III)
    Other

Occupational therapy
    A home visit was done on ....
    by the following paramedical staff:

    Aids arranged and expected delivery date:

    Area OT involved:

    Any follow-up visits arranged:

Physiotherapy
    Mobility on discharge:
    Wheelchair issued:
    OP physiotherapy arranged:
    Community physiotherapist contacted:
    Any follow-up visits arranged:

Family/friends and support:

9

Management of the upper limb amputee

INTRODUCTION

Prostheses for the upper limb amputee are required following amputation for trauma, amputation for disease and for congenital limb deficiency. Amputations for trauma follow road traffic accidents, industrial and farming accidents and include burns and brachial plexus lesions. Amputations for disease are due to vascular conditions such as Raynaud's phenomenon, Buerger's disease, diabetes and malignancy. Congenital limb deficiencies may be due to a failure of formation or differentiation of parts at an early stage of pregnancy, duplication, over or undergrowth, congenital construction band syndrome or generalized skeletal abnormalities.

Upper limb amputation is less common in the UK than lower limb amputation by a ratio of approximately 1:26 and the male:female ratio is 8:1 (Thornberry, 1986, personal communication). In 1982 there were 203 upper limb amputees referred to limb fitting centres in England, Wales and Northern Ireland for prosthetic care. In 1985 this figure was 145 and the levels of loss were as follows: 14 about the shoulder, 60 above the elbow, 4 elbow disarticulations, 37 below the elbow and four at the wrist and the remainder (26) above the hand (Ham *et al.*, 1989). The number of upper limb amputees has fallen because of better Health and Safety practices at the work place. Forty per cent of all primary upper limb referrals to the prosthetic centres in the UK are for congenital deficiency. Referrals between the ages of 10 and 17 years are generally for trauma or malignant disease and in adults over 18 years, the largest group, the cause is generally industrial or road traffic accidents.

In Denmark a similar number of upper limb amputations were seen over a 6 year period (Andersen-Ranberg and Ebskov, 1988). The majority of above-elbow amputees reported were for vascular disease or malignancy and the hand amputations were for vascular disease, malignancy, infection and trauma. In the Third World the figures are different. In India and Hong Kong the ratio of upper limb to lower limb is 2:1 and in Burma 4:1.

Therefore, in the west, the upper limb amputee is generally either a child, an adolescent or a working adult, all with productive years ahead and an active contribution to make in society. It is therefore important that the highest level of function is achieved for these patients as soon as possible and early referral to an experienced prosthetic centre is essential (Durance and O'Shea, 1988). In some cases of disease such as malignancy or vascular conditions, the patients will be seen and treated pre-operatively. If so this will include counselling, physical exercises and an introduction to the team and appropriate prosthetic equipment. For the traumatic cases this may not be possible.

PRE-PROSTHETIC TRAINING PHASE

The upper limb amputee experiences psychological loss which is often greater than following loss of a leg (see Chapter 10). The hands and arms have both a social and functional purpose. They are used for expression, communication, affection, manual dexterity, sexual identity, work, recreation and provide the individual with a total body image. In communication the upper limb comes only second to the face as a means of non-verbal communication. The loss of an upper limb therefore produces feelings of inadequacy, especially if the dominant arm/hand is lost and these patients require much psychological support and encouragement from the whole team. However, this can be helped by teaching the patient as soon as possible how to become independent, especially for personal activities which will help to regain their self-esteem. Help with adapting clothes, by adding velcro for example, and feeding may also be necessary, especially for the bilateral amputee. The therapist will help the patient appreciate the usefulness of the stump and maintain neurophysiological movement patterns and so prevent one-handed practices (Eyre, 1979). It is important that patients are given an early realistic picture of the appearance and function of the prothesis that is to be prescribed. The prosthesis should be described as a tool for function and cosmesis and it should be emphasized that it will never be functionally equivalent to the part that has been lost. For some patients the main concern is function, for others it is cosmesis, for the majority it is a combination of these two factors.

At the time of amputation, the patient and his family need support from all the staff. The therapist can help them come to terms with the appearance of the stump by handling the stump during therapy which also helps to desensitize it and by using treatments such as massage, which helps to prevent scar adhesions forming. Upper limb amputees, like the lower limb amputee, are also likely to experience phantom sensation and pain (Chapter 7).

During this period, the management programme will include physical exercise, psychological support, oedema control and stump care. The physiotherapist, occupational therapist, nurse, social worker and possibly the clinical psychologist will therefore work closely together as a team with the surgeon, doctors and prosthetist. The patient will be assessed, which will include the following information: aetiology and onset, age, dominance, other medical problems, level of independence, range of motion, muscle power, skin cover, muscle bulk, state of uninvolved limbs' operative revisions, phantom pain, control sites and pain. The patient's expections will be noted, as well as the social support he has, his hobbies, educational background and his employment. This information is used to ensure that the correct prescription for each individual patient is achieved. Physically the therapists will work together to strengthen the shoulder girdle and remaining muscles and maintain joint mobility. Strong shoulder girdle actions which include the scapula and especially the movement of protraction, are essential for prosthetic use and contractures should be avoided through advice, positioning and exercise. An early active exercise programme will help to increase the circulation and therefore reduce oedema in the stump. Resistance is added later as the patient is able to tolerate it. A light dressing is usually applied immediately post-operatively and then traditional or modified stump bandaging or a stump shrinker once the wound is healed. As the patient improves and the stump becomes less sensitive, more active and resisted exercise should be carried out.

Upper limb amputees have a tendency to flex towards the amputated side and lose their arm swing during walking as it is held rigidly to the trunk. Scoliosis has also been reported (Durance and O'Shea, 1988) but these postural deformities can be avoided by balance retraining, active exercise and educating the patient. The future prosthesis is made as light as possible (average 1.3 kg) and therefore does not provide the weight to assist with body symmetry.

At approximately 3–10 days after the amputation, a leather gauntlet is applied to the stump into which objects are added to encourage a two-handed approach to general activities and avoid general stiffness. For the below-elbow patient, objects, for example utensils, and for the above-elbow patient, a bat for general exercises, may be added (Mendez, 1985). When the dominant hand is lost the patient will need to be re-educated to transfer dominance to the opposite side and also helped in co-ordination and skilful movement (Heger, 1982).

Once the stump is healing well the patient is referred to a specialist upper limb clinic team. At the initial visit the patient and their family will meet the prosthetic team members and aspects of amputation, loss and future management will be discussed. The care of the stump, the different types of prosthesis, the terminology and the technology of prosthesis, are also discussed as appropriate (Cooper, 1989, personnal communication). It is important that the patient and their family have the opportunity to ask questions and give their opinions at this time.

PROSTHETIC TRAINING PHASE

There are three aims in this phase:

1. to teach the function and potential of the artificial limb;
2. to gain the maximum usefulness of the artificial limb in connection with work, independence and recreation; and
3. to help restore morale (Eyre, 1979).

The comfort and fit of the prosthesis are important and the stump should be checked regularly to ensure that no pressure areas have developed, especially with patients who lack sensation. Following the prosthetic fitting, the patient is taught how to care for the prosthesis, how to put on and take off the limb and how to use it functionally. For patients who wear a shoulder harness, a vest for comfort and hygiene is generally worn.

There are three stages to training:

1. control of the limb – the patient learns how the controls the mechanisms of the individual prosthesis work;
2. use of the limb in bilateral activity – the patient exercises using the limb so he becomes aware of its benefits; and
3. use of appliances – once the patient has become aware of the usefulness of the limb, appliances for leisure and work activities are introduced.

Exercises are selected to increase the dexterity and speed of prosthetic use (Heger, 1982). The training periods should be arranged on a full-time basis on consecutive days, for as long a period each day as possible. For the below-elbow amputee this is generally for one week and for the above-elbow amputee for approximately two weeks. Once the patient is confident he can continue to practise in his own environment. Handling of the prosthesis is an ongoing learning process and the purpose of training is to learn the basic functions of the prosthesis. Double amputees can take between three months and a year to retrain (Eyre, 1979).

Training with the split hook is practised using, for example, peg games. The difficulty of the tasks are increased to involve different objects, shapes, sizes and textures of increasing complexity. Learning to operate the elbow mechanism automatically demands a great deal of patience and determination and is often practised initially in front of a mirror to help the patient see the necessary physical movement (Eyre, 1979). Only 54% of patients in a recent survey received training and they all requested more, especially for leisure activities. It was found that the above-elbow level of amputation had a bigger impact on the vocational aspect than the below-elbow level amputee (Durance and O'Shea, 1988).

A person's prosthetic needs change as they go through life and therefore prosthetic changes need to be made appropriately.

LEVELS OF LOSS AND THE PROSTHETIC REPLACEMENT

Prostheses aim to replace the missing part by restoring the amputee's body image and by being functionally useful and cosmetically acceptable. Upper limb prostheses are designed to incorporate a method of suspension, a socket to provide the interface between the patient and the prosthesis, a joint mechanism if appropriate, the mechanical hand or terminal device which is the main functional component and the skeletal element between the two which exists to position the hand or terminal device in space and a power source or control system.

The *suspension* may be self-suspending as with modern lower limb prostheses or it may include a harness system. The *socket* may be made of leather or modern materials and may either be a total contact cup socket or self-suspending. The *joint mechanism*, for example the elbow, may be internal or external depending upon the length of the remanent limb and the room available. The *skeletal element* or infill will vary in length, depending upon the size of the remaining limb, as with the below-knee prosthesis and its cosmesis may vary. The *power source* may be body powered by a harness and shoulder movements, electrically or with gas. The *control system* may be by loop and cord, pulley, a servo-electric or myoelectric system. The *terminal device* may be a cosmetic hand, split hook or a specific functional device such as a spade holder.

The surgical principles described in Chapter 5 also apply to the upper limb.

Partial hand

Partial hand amputations are usually due to trauma and involve the loss of one or more digits or there may also be loss of part of the carpus skeleton area. Function may be improved by surgery to the hand remnant, for example pollicization or toe transplantation. Although the surgical procedures are different, the functional aims are the same. A simple opposition plate may be supplied to restore palmar grip for holding a knife and fork, for example, or a gloved hand may be indicated for cosmetic appearances only. A functional prosthesis which offers a weak pinch grip on flexion of the partial hand remnant has been developed at the Princess Margaret Rose Hospital in Edinburgh.

Wrist disarticulation

This level is generally due to a traumatic amputation or a congenital limb deficiency. A leather gauntlet which provides an attachment for a terminal device and a cosmetic glove hand may be all that these patients require. To allow pronation and supination to take place, a split forearm socket may be used (Mendez, 1985). If the patient is carrying out heavy work a prosthesis similar to that supplied for a below-elbow stump will be necessary.

Below elbow

Below-elbow prostheses are supplied for congenital deformity or following surgical amputation. For a planned amputation the stump should be 17 cm below the olecrannon process of the elbow to provide a good lever and 4 cm above the wrist joint line to allow a 'wrist rotary' or terminal device attachment to be accommodated. There are two types of prosthesis for this level. The cup socket which may use a figure of eight harness around the shoulders for suspension and an operational cord to activate the terminal device or it may be suspended from an upper arm corset with two side steels or the supracondylar socket which is self-suspending with no additional straps, or socks, but full extension of the elbow is lost. A lightweight 'one piece' arm may be supplied for cosmetic reasons only. With the body powered arm, the terminal device is operated by protrusion of the opposite shoulder which activates the single loop appendage which transmits the power through the operational cord which is threaded down the prosthesis. The myoelectric prosthesis, originally developed for this level of loss, may also be prescribed. Regular stump inspections should be a part of training.

The prosthesis includes a 'wrist rotary' into which terminal devices are inserted. The most common device is the split hook which provides a high degree of manipulative skill and function. It is opened actively and closed passively once the tension is released. The strength of the grip can be altered by changing the resistance bands. As the band is increased, greater body power is required to activate the device. Other terminal devices are available, for example the floating spoon, universal tool holder, billiard cue holder and rest, spade grip, golfing appliance, quick grip pliers and a fishing rod holder. (Companies will make special devices for an amputee with a special interest.) Alternatively a cosmetic mechanical hand may be chosen. It has limited function but provides cosmetic replacement. All patients in the UK are provided with a cosmetic hand.

Elbow disarticulation

This is not an elective site for amputation due to the cosmetic and functional shortcomings of the prosthesis. External hinged elbow joints are required which are both bulky and unreliable and there is not space for an internal elbow mechanism.

Above elbow

Surgical amputation at this level is generally performed for trauma or malignancy. The site of amputation is ideally 7–10 cm above the olecrannon process of the elbow or at the junction of the upper two thirds and lower third of the humerus. The longer the length of the residual stump the better the control the patient has of the prosthesis, but consideration should be given to elbow flexion occurring at an anatomical level. The elected site allows for the incorporation of a rotary device above the artificial joint offering internal and external rotation of the forearm component. The prosthesis consists of an arm section, moulded to fit over the stump and point of the shoulder, an elbow unit, forearm wrist unit and detachable hand. The suspension is around the amputee's back and opposite shoulder by a harness. Flexion of the elbow and gripping is achieved by protraction of the shoulder girdle and humeral flexion. Locking of the elbow unit is achieved by depression and extension of the glenohumeral joint, a trick movement which is often difficult to learn (Cooper, 1989, personal communication). Some patients find it easier to place the elbow in the desired position of flexion and lock it using their good arm. The artificial elbow joint has a lock which engages in chosen positions of flexion and extension. Terminal devices are available as for the below-elbow level and the wrist unit has a push-button device to remove and lock the terminal device.

Shoulder disarticulation

This level of amputation is generally performed for malignancy or trauma. The clavicle and acromion are trimmed to leave a rounded contour which is better to fit a prosthesis and reduces pressure. For this level a prosthesis that is cosmetic, functional and resembles that of the above elbow but has a wider embracing socket is used. Hinged or rigid shoulders may be supplied, the hinged type being preferred as it allows a limited amount of free movement when the wearer changes position and therefore provides less of a drag on the body (Robertson, 1978). The elbow mechanism is locked passively by the remaining hand but it is functionally limited, only being used for steading or holding down objects.

Forequarter

This level of amputation is rarely performed but when necessary it is generally for neoplastic disease. The clavicle and scapula are removed and a simple cosmetic cap is commonly provided to a cast of the shoulder remnant or upper thorax for cosmetic appearance in clothing. This is initially made from plastazote by the therapist and then by the prosthetist. Often a sleeve filler made from foam with a cosmetic hand is provided (Mendez, 1985).

CONGENITAL LIMB DEFICIENCY

Congenital limb deficiency accounts for 40% of all referrals to the prosthetic centres in the UK. The ratio of congenital upper limb to lower limb is 5:1. In the past the recording of congenital absence varied between clinicians. Today, following work by the International Society of Prosthetics and Orthotics, an International Standard is available to record such deficiencies. Loss or absence is described either in the longitudinal or transverse plane and as being either total or partial (ISO 8548/9). Such children should be referred to the prosthetic centre early so that the parents and family can meet the team and start to understand the rehabilitation process. The programme should be carefully explained to the parents, who are generally under considerable stress and feeling guilty about the child's deficiency (Chapter 10). Early involvement of the parents helps the future prosthetic compliance of the child as it is the parents, especially the mother, who acts as co-therapist in the training programmes (Eyre, 1979).

Initially a one piece cosmetic arm is fitted, a sleeve filler, when the child is approximately 6 months old. This is changed as the child grows to ensure that the prosthesis is suitable for use when sitting balance begins. Once manipulation skills develop, at approximately 18 months, the first working prosthesis is provided. This is generally a split hook, which, although functionally effective, is poor in appearance and the parents may need help and support to become accustomed to it. The functional scope and potential for the split hook should be explained to the parents (Eyre, 1979). The child is reviewed at the prosthetic clinic every 3 months when the prosthesis is changed according to growth and further training started as the child's skills develop. When the child starts to attend the nursery or school, it may be necessary for therapist to link up with the teacher to ensure continuity of activities and to explain the child's limitations and potential (Mendez, 1985).

Children with multiple limb deficiencies have many functional problems. There are also more stresses placed on the family than in cases of a single limb deficiency. The reduced body surface area and the extra covering necessary when limbs are worn, leads to an increase in sweating in the remaining limbs. Prostheses may be provided but they take a great deal of effort and energy to use.

MYOELECTRIC CONTROL

The first published account of myoelectric control was in 1948 (Reiter, 1948). Research and development continued in a number of countries during the 1960s and the first systems were clinically available in the 1970s. Myoelectric control uses the electrical activity of a contracting muscle as the control system to work the prosthesis (Scott and Parker, 1988). A rechargeable battery is also included in the device for energy storage and the amputees are given four batteries which are recharged at night.

Myoelectric prostheses are generally fitted to children between the ages of three and a half and four and a half years but reports of successful fitting at 18 months are found. This type of prosthesis has an intimate fit, is comfortable to wear and provides freedom from harnessing and because of this and its design, it is more cosmetically acceptable. Functional activities above the shoulder are also possible. It is essential that patients using myoelectric prostheses are given adequate information and training at the time of fitting (Herberts *et al.*, 1980). Training usually takes 2 days with a possible further session a couple of weeks later. The therapist initially trains the parents or guardians who in turn train the children. Any problems should be noticed as soon as possible to enable there to be a continuity of use and limb wearing.

The conventional or body-operated prosthesis is lighter, less expensive and more reliable and it allows greater activity of movement at the elbow and forearm (Weaver *et al.*, 1988). However, the higher the level of the amputation the greater is the effort required to work the prosthesis. It is for the higher levels of amputation that the greatest benefits will be seen in the future. A myoelectric hand has also been successfully applied together with a conventional elbow lock to amputees with above-elbow loss where suitable electrode sites have been identified. The myoelectric hand activates opposition of the thumb towards flexion of the index and middle fingers in a three point pinch grip.

Electrically powered elbow units are now available, for example the Utah elbow and the Servo system.

REFERENCES

Andersen-Ranberg, F. and Ebskov, B. (1988) Major upper extremity amputation in Denmark. *Acta Orthop. Scand.*, **59**, 321–322.

Durance, J.P. and O'Shea, B.J. (1988) Upper limb amputees: a clinic profile. *Int. Disabil. Studies*, **10**, 68–72.

Eyre, N.C. (1979) Rehabilitation of the upper limb amputee. *Physiotherapy*, **65**, 9–12.

Ham, R.O., Luff, R. and Roberts, V.C. (1989) A 5-year review of referrals for prosthetic treatment in England, Wales and Northern Ireland 1981–85. *Health Trends*, **21**, 2–5.

Heger, H. (1982) Training of upper extremity amputees, in *Rehabilitation Management of Amputees* (ed. S.N. Banerjee), pp. 255–295. Rehabilitation Medicine Library, Baltimore.

Herberts, P., Körner, L., Caine, K. and Wensby, L. (1980) Rehabilitation of unilateral below-elbow amputees with myoelectric prostheses. *Scand. J. Rehab. Med.*, **12**, 123–128.

Mendez, A. (1985) Upper limb amputation and congenital limb deficiency, in *Physiotherapy for Amputees. The Roehampton Approach*, Churchill Livingstone, Edinburgh, pp. 222–247.

Reiter, R. (1948) Eine neue Electrokunsthand. *Grenzgebiete der Medizin*, **1**, 133–135.

Robertson, E. (1978) Types of prostheses, in *Rehabilitation of Arm Amputees and Limb Deficient Children*, pp. 30–40. Baillière Tindall, London.

Scott, R.N. and Parker, P.A. (1988) Myoelectric prostheses; state of the art. *J. Med. Eng. Tech.*, **12**, 143–151.

Weaver, S.A., Lange, L.R. and Vogt, V.M. (1988) Comparison of myoelectric and conventional prostheses for adolescent amputees. *Am. J. Occup. Ther.*, **42**, 87–91.

10

Psychological and social aspects of amputation

PSYCHOLOGICAL ASPECTS

The loss of a limb is a stressful event in anyone's life, producing emotional and psychological disturbances. How the patient reacts to amputation is very individual and chiefly depends upon their personality. However, other factors also play a part; the nature of the current experience, their previous life experiences, their expectations and attitude to disability and the support given by their family and society. Often patients showing the best early acceptance of amputation may not be the ones who come to terms with the situation best in the long term. They may later show a delayed depressive reaction.

Bereavement

All patients who have an amputation will bereave or mourn the loss of their limb, the natural process that occurs following a loss and they will all feel grief, the personal experience of loss. These are normal reactions by which we begin to meet the loss that has occurred, whether it is an amputation or divorce, miscarriage or the death of a loved one (Parkes, 1972). Bereavement is not a state but is a process which takes place over time and a number of overlapping 'phases' or 'tasks'. Some authors call these processes 'phases' (Parkes and Napier, 1970) and others call them 'tasks' as they are something which the mourner passes through and can take action on, whereas the word 'phase' is thought to be more passive (Worden, 1983a).

There are four tasks involved in the bereavement process:

1. to accept the reality of the loss as it is often hard to believe the finality of the loss initially;
2. to experience the pain of grief which must be worked through if the pain is not to be carried with the bereaved person throughout their life;
3. to adjust to an environment in which the loss is missing; and
4. to withdraw emotional energy and re-invest it into other activities or relationships (Worden, 1983b).

The normal grief reaction

Whilst there are large individual differences in the way people cope with loss and bereavement, there is a main pattern which the grieving process follows. Three main stages can be identified and they may overlap but they serve as a useful guide to identifying where in the grieving process a person is at a particular time (Worden, 1983a).

Stage 1: Numbness

This usually lasts 2–3 days after the loss and helps the person to disregard the loss temporarily. At this time people need help, often with the simplest decisions.

Stage 2: Despair

This is a very painful stage, involving peaks of anguish and distress. The features of this phase fall into four general categories, though not all of them will be seen in any one person:

1. feelings of sadness, anger and frustration, guilt and self-reproach, anxiety, loneliness, fatigue, helplessness, shock, pining, emancipation, relief or numbness;
2. physical sensations of which the most common are hollowness in the stomach, tightness in the chest and throat, dry mouth, lack of energy and depersonalization – 'nothing feeling real';
3. cognitions or thought patterns of disbelief, confusion, preoccupation or hallucinations; and
4. behaviours such as sleep and appetite disturbances, social withdrawal, dreams, absent-mindedness, avoiding reminders, crying or restless overactivity.

Stage 3: Recovery

During this stage the person gradually begins to put life together again, adapting and rebuilding it to accommodate the changes needed in the light of their loss. It is impossible to give a normal or average time for completion of the grieving process as so many factors influence the individual. The closeness of the relationship with the deceased is a crucial factor and for a very close relationship it is generally felt that resolution is unlikely to occur within a year. A good benchmark is when the person is able to think of the deceased or lost limb without the painful wrenching quality experienced earlier. Bereavement and grieving is therefore a long-term process (Ham and Kerfoot, 1989).

The atypical grief reaction

There are three characteristics which can help to distinguish between a normal and an atypical grief reaction.

1. A prolonged reaction, where after many years the third stage, recovery, is not seen.
2. A delayed reaction. This often relates to a persistent denial of the reality and finality of the loss and a difficulty in moving into Stage 2.
3. Increased and persistent feelings of guilt and self blame. If unresolved these may contribute to a depressive illness.

Determinants of grief

Although there are large individual differences, there are also certain factors that can alert staff to particular patients who may have difficulty resolving their grief following amputation. These factors may be in the patient's personal history, for example a childhood loss and other recent losses or a life crisis, especially if it occurred in the previous two years. Knowledge of how the patient coped with these losses is a useful indicator and also if he has a past medical history of depression and mental illness. At the time of amputation, women and the young tend to be more susceptible and they will therefore require more support. Cultural practices and family reactions and the way the amputation occurred also need to be taken into consideration. After the amputation, staff should note whether the patient has social support or is isolated. They should also note if the amputee gains from the amputation, perhaps for example socially or financially (Worden, 1983a).

Counselling the bereaved

Most health care professionals have the skill and sensitivity to help those experiencing a normal grief reaction to bereavement. They can help by listening to amputees and giving them time to talk and by acknowledging their special loss and the feelings they are experiencing, by not denying or rushing their feelings, pointing out actions of avoidance and self blame and helping them to make simple decisions. In addition, being able to identify those who are experiencing serious problems and referring them for specialist help and grief therapy is of great value (Ham and Kerfoot, 1989).

Surgery

The patient's adjustment starts pre-operatively and the fears and uncertainty felt can be averted with adequate preparation (Parkes and Napier, 1970). In applicable cases, notably vascular disease, cancer and some traumatic cases, the patient should be warned early that amputation is a probability. This keeps the patient informed and stops the feeling that amputation is a treatment of failure rather than a life-saving, reconstructive (Friedman, 1978; Bradway et al., 1984) or positive step forward. The surgeon should inform the patient of the reason the operation is necessary and give a brief or lay explanation of the procedure, explaining about the pain, the analgesics and how recovery will take place. Effective communication prior to surgery has been found by many authors to reduce post-operative complications and analgesic requirements, both of which help early discharge (Richards and McDonald, 1985).

A realistic future for the individual patient should be discussed following team discussions and the surgeon should avoid telling the patient 'you will be almost normal after we fit you with an artificial leg'. The principal family members should also be kept informed by the hospital team and they should be welcomed into the ward. The amputation should only be performed when it has been agreed by the patient and discussed with their immediate family. Once the decision has been made, it should be carried out as soon as possible, allowing time for the patient to be fully assessed and treated by the appropriate team members (Chapter 6). It is also helpful for an amputee of a similar age, level of amputation and personality to talk to the prospective amputee pre-operatively (Ham and Kerfoot, 1987).

Rehabilitation

Group treatment sessions for the amputee have been found to be most successful. The new amputee meets the more experienced patient who has much advice to offer of how to cope with practical and emotional problems. The motivation and experience of the therapists is important, as is their attitude towards amputation and rehabilitation and the way they convey this to the patient. An active rehabilitation programme gives the patient less time to dwell on fears and anxieties and less time to feel depressed before achieving more positive rehabilitation activities. The individual amputee's progress will depend on how they cope and adjust to the loss. Success will depend on age, medical condition, motivation, family and social support. Therapists must teach the patients to become independent and avoid dependence 'even though it helps the therapist to feel needed' (Friedman, 1978).

Returning home is a critical period and pre-discharge home visits are essential so that the problems are brought back to the hospital and solved before the patient is discharged (Ham and Kerfoot, 1987). Domicilary services for these patients should be arranged as a matter of routine, rather than leaving the patient or their relatives to organize these alone (Froggatt and Mawby, 1981). Therapists and nurses spend a great deal of time with the amputee so they must be prepared and be knowledgeable enough to answer the amputee's questions. During the operative period, the patient becomes dependent on the staff. As the patient gets better and gradually becomes more independent, staff will notice that their complaints increase (Friedman, 1978).

The homunculus in the brain contains a 'working model' of each limb. It is therefore not surprising that the physical amputation of the limb does not remove this 'working model' (Parkes, 1972). It is therefore important that patients are warned of the feeling of their limb or phantom sensation (see Chapter 7) in the first post-operative weeks. These feelings will help the patient during prosthetic use and walking.

Prosthetics

Following amputation the patient loses his body image (Parkes and Napier, 1970) and an artificial limb or prosthesis helps to restore this and conceal the new disability. This is especially important for women. Some authors feel it is essential for the patient to experience a period of mourning before the prosthesis is fitted (Goldberg, 1984) but that it should not be delayed for long, as walking is a positive activity for the patient and prolonged delay can reinforce negative attitudes.

The patient's adjustment to the prosthesis has been found to depend upon their own personal adjustment to amputation. The less trouble the patient experiences with the prosthesis, the fewer emotional problems will be exhibited and the better social integration will be. Patients who abandon their prostheses repeatedly saying that they do not fit will continue to abandon them, so there is no point in represcribing for these cases. Some patients are critical of the prosthesis as it does not closely mimic the normal limb. These patients are highly vulnerable to the attitudes and emotions of others (Friedman, 1978) and appropriate help and counselling will be necessary. Patients must be told and shown that prostheses are not like normal limbs and this will help them to adjust to using the new limb.

Upper limb amputees

The upper limb amputees find it harder to adjust to amputation than the lower limb amputees as the arm and hand are important in social interaction and the prosthesis is more noticeable and socially less acceptable. They often hide their artificial hand under a newspaper or perhaps travel on public transport at the same time so that they see the same people and not new faces who stare. It is important that the upper limb stump is touched, especially by loved ones, but also by staff.

Amputation for congenital defects

When amputation has been performed for a congenital deformity, it is important that staff also treat the parents, as they need immediate help to repair the damage to their self-esteem and marital bond. This damage is the result of the guilt, rage and despair that the creation of an imperfect infant has caused (Kohl, 1984). This will ensure that the child will then develop with a positive sense of self and rehabilitation will be successful. Many of the child's close family should also have contact with the medical and rehabilitation team to help this process. The emotional reaction is felt by both parents but especially by the mother and suicidal or psychotic breakdowns are frequent in the months following the birth (Friedman, 1978).

Amputation after trauma

The traumatic amputee mourns for the lost part of their body and their physical, emotional and social worlds have to be re-established. It is best if the emotional needs can become part of the treatment plan. If the trauma has occurred to a young child, the parents will feel guilty and need help. The young child will regress emotionally and lose previously mastered milestones. The adult traumatic case will feel fear and anger at losing their independence, and having to rely on others. They may also feel guilty because of the way the limb was lost. They will also have to redefine every personal and working relationship, and only if the result is positive and constructive will they find a new sense of self (Kohl, 1984). Amputees who have managerial or professional jobs will have fewer problems in continuing to work than those of the lower socio-economic groups who rely on their physical state for employment.

Amputations for disease

Patients with arterial disease or cancer may initially feel great relief when their pain is removed. These patients have generally been ill for some time prior to the operation and have not been as active as usual. Often the numerous operations the patient has experienced make the prosthesis less cosmetically acceptable as it does not fully restore their body image. For the elderly patient the possible move to a nursing home, where they are unable to cope physically, is often more painful than the amputation itself. Such a move is linked with rejection and exclusion from the family and society and is regarded as a place where one awaits death (Kohl, 1984). Cancer patients also have to cope with this fear of death.

GENERAL

Most amputees resent sympathy but have a need for empathy. They feel they have lost the ability to relate psychologically, socially, sexually and vocationally and this inhibits them most in their recovery. The younger amputee will in general adjust well. They will, however, share their feelings of inferiority of being 'incomplete' with other amputees and this is especially common with women. Self-help groups prove to be invaluable. For the older patient it is more difficult as they have less psychological resilience, are often chronically depressed and are less physically able to withstand major surgery (Parkes and Napier, 1970). Some patients, however, become emotionally destroyed by amputation and lose a will to live or fail to thrive. Cole Porter, for example, never wrote another hit song following his amputation. The financial and emotional burdens are as great for the amputee as for any disabled person.

SOCIAL ASPECTS

The social aspects of work with amputees are predominantly covered by the *hospital social worker*. In the UK social workers are employed by local authorities and have statutory duties in the areas of mental health, child care, the elderly and the chronically sick and disabled. They act for patients by liaising with the statutory bodies, the local authority social service and housing departments, the Department of Social Security, the police, the Community Health Services and the Disablement Resettlement Officer, for example. They also liaise with voluntary bodies, such as Age Concern, the British Legion, specialist health groups, churches, local organizations, ethnic and support groups, as well as with other members of the hospital team to negotiate and achieve better results for the patient.

Social workers in this country advise patients on which welfare rights or benefits they may be entitled to: sickness, invalidity benefit, retirement pension, income support, housing benefit, attendance allowance, mobility allowance, invalid care allowance, severe disablement allowance and possibly the industrial injuries scheme (Ham and Kerfoot, 1987). They will also advise and assist the amputee on other resources to which they may be entitled, for example the bus pass, disabled driver's disc, Dial a Ride, Taxicard scheme, exemption from vehicle excise duty and Mobility Allowance (Roberts, 1982), Motability, ethnic switchboards and charity organizations such as RADAR and Disabled Living Foundation. They are often regarded as a door to door library of information (Sherwood, 1984).

The role of the social worker is generally to relieve and prevent social distress, to help with social and personal problems linked to illness, age or disability and to work towards the emotional well-being of the patient and strengthening of their relationships. Social workers will counsel patients regarding grief and loss and help them make full use of hospital treatment and return to their own environment with as much independence as possible. They advise on nursing homes and private or voluntary residential homes, but the responsibility for these placements is with the patient and their family or with various placement schemes that may be established in any particular hospital. Social workers are responsible for assessing patients for local authorities (or Part III) residential homes and, where appropriate, arranging such a placement.

Referrals to the social worker are made by the patient, a relative or the staff. The referring person should, however, have informed the patient that the referral has been made and the reason for it. Often the initial presenting problem may be straightforward, for example home help or meals on wheels, but it may indicate a greater need for involvement and assistance. The social worker is said to be someone who is prepared to be on equal terms with the disabled person and not someone who hides behind a professional screen. Much of social work with disabled people is about encouraging them to make full use of their own resources and rekindle former skills and develop new ones so that the individual takes control of their own life (Sherwood, 1984).

The social worker is also actively involved with the amputee's discharge and this discharge planning starts on admission. Discharge planning aims to prepare the patient and their family physiologically and psychologically for the transfer home, promote the highest level of independence for the patient and their family, provide continuity of care between the hospital and the community and make the transfer smooth (Jupp and Simms, 1986). A discharge date one week ahead is generally given to the amputee and Fridays are avoided for those patients who require much social service support.

SOCIAL SERVICES

The social circumstances of many patients, especially the elderly, are profoundly influenced by the practical aspects of rehabilitation. Social workers are involved in the acute stage, supporting and counselling the patient and their relatives and they also refer to and work with the supportive services of the community, notably the social services.

Each local authority in the UK provides services to the elderly and disabled through the social service department. Throughout the country, there is much unevenness in how much support and the number of services that all provide (Rudinger, 1979). In some areas support and services are means tested, in others they are free. The frequency of the service, for example meals on wheels and home helps, and the amount of money spent on luncheon clubs and house adaptations also vary throughout the UK.

In some areas free bath boards are given to the disabled, in others they are not given 'unless there is a medical reason for the patient to have a bath' (Filby, 1989, personal communication). Once the patient receives help from the social service department he may be placed on the local register of the disabled. Social service departments commonly provide the following services: meals on wheels, home help, aids and adaptations, housing adaptations, day centres, lunch clubs, chiropody, hairdressing, telephones, radios, alarm systems, visiting library services, holiday homes and assistance, financial help and information about local concessions, for example reduced transport fares and residential homes (Part III) for the elderly.

REFERENCES

Bradway, J.K., Malone, J.M., Lacy, J., Leal, J.M. and Poole, J. (1984) Psychological adaptation to amputation: an overview. *Othotics Prosthetics*, **38**, 46–50.

Friedman, L.W. (1978) *The Psychological Rehabilitation of the Amputee*. Thomas, London.

Froggatt, D. and Mawby, R.T. (1981) Surviving an amputation. *Soc. Sci. Med.*, **15E**, 123–128.

Goldberg, R.T. (1984) New trends in the rehabilitation of lower extremity amputees. *Rehabilitation Literature*, **45**, 2–11.

Ham, R. and Kerfoot, S. (1987) *Recovering from Amputation – the Dulwich Way*. King's College School of Medicine and Dentistry and Camberwell Health Authority.

Ham, R. and Kerfoot, S. (1989) *Information for Staff Dealing with Patients Undergoing Amputation*. Carters, Westbury, Wilts.

Ham, R., Regan, J.M. and Roberts, V.C. (1987) Evaluation of introducing the team approach to the care of the amputee: the Dulwich study. *Prosthet. Orthot. Int.*, **11**, 25–30.

Jupp, M. and Simms, S. (1986) Going home. *Nursing Times*, 1 October, 40–42.

Kohl, S.J. (1984) Emotional coping with amputation, in *Rehabilitation Psychology* (ed. D. Krueger), Aspen Publications, London, pp. 273–282.

Parkes, C.M. (1972) Components of the reaction to loss of a limb, spouse or home. *J. Psychosom. Res.*, **16**, 343–349.

Parkes, C.M. and Napier, M.M. (1970) Psychiatric sequellae of amputation. *Br. J. Hosp. Med.*, **7**, 610–614.

Richards, J. and McDonald, P. (1985) Doctor–patient communication in surgery. *J. R. Soc. Med.*, **78**, 922–924.

Roberts, G.S. (1982) The Mobility Allowance – a review of the initial 5 years. *Health Trends*, **14**, 13–15.

Rudinger, E. (1979) *Coping with Disablement*. Open University, Milton Keynes, pp. 1–7.

Sherwood, E. (1984) The Social Worker: a community resource. *Contact*, winter, p. 39.

Worden, J.W. (1983a) Normal grief reactions: Uncomplicated mourning, in *Grief Counselling and Grief Therapy*, Tavistock, London, pp. 19–33.

Worden, J.W. (1983b) Attachment, loss and the task of mourning, in *Grief Counselling and Grief Therapy*, Tavistock, London, pp. 7–18.

11

The prosthetic service in the UK

HISTORICAL INTRODUCTION

Before 1914, the number of amputees in the UK was small and the surgical mortality rate high. Those who survived amputation generally become mobile using crutches and few had artificial limbs as they could not afford to buy them. During the First World War (1914–1918) a 25 bedded hospital was opened for war amputees. This was in a converted Queen Anne mansion known as Roehampton House in London. Queen Mary was patron and the hospital became known as one of 'Queen Mary's Convalescent Auxiliary Hospitals' for limbless soldiers and sailors. Other similar centres also opened at this time throughout the country but as the artificial limb suppliers were not located near to the hospital, amputees who needed limbs visited these craftsmen in their limb shops. With the influx of amputees during the war, these shops gradually moved into the grounds at Roehampton and the other centres to be nearer the patients.

In 1916 the relevant government department, the Ministry of Pensions, became responsible for supplying limbs to all war pensioners free of charge. There were many small artificial limb suppliers at the time, notably Charles A. Blatchford, Gustov Ernst (who later evolved the company into Vessa Ltd) and two American companies, Rowley's and Hangers (later to become J. E. Hanger & Co.). In 1919, a government Departmental Committee was appointed to advise the Minister of 'any improvements that were thought possible in the supplying, fitting and maintaining of artificial limbs to the war amputees, trying to minimise delays'. Before the war, amputees would visit a limbmaker who was paid privately and a surgeon's certificate was obtained at a later date stating that the limb was suitable. With the

influx of war amputees, the practice was changed. The limb was prescribed by the surgeon who then supervised its fitting and finally passed it when it was acceptable (English and Gregory Dean, 1980).

Centres had been established in London, Liverpool, Manchester, Leeds, Birmingham, Belfast and Cardiff during the war and others at Aberdeen, Newcastle and Norwich were established soon afterwards. By the end of the war, 28 000 artificial legs and 12 000 artificial arms had been supplied by the government through the Ministry of Pensions. The basis of the prosthetic service in Britain that was to last until the 1980s, was now established. Surgeons supervised the limb prescription and fitting, some component parts were standardized and each level of amputation had one or two designs of limb that were appropriate for that level. Staff, both medical and administrative, became directly responsible to the Ministry of Pensions and responsible for other services related to the war pensioner, for example the orthotic or surgical appliance service and the issuing of invalid tricycles which also came under this Ministry. The civilian amputee's lot had however not improved. They continued to use 'peg leg' designs or to regain their mobility by using crutches. When they did receive an artificial limb, this was funded by either a charity or from a private source (McColl, 1986).

With improvements in surgical techniques, care and drugs, the Second World War (1935–1945) did not produce such an influx of amputees as did the First World War. By the end of the war, 45 000 limbless war pensioners were being cared for by the Ministry of Pensions and the prosthetic company Hangers had the government monopoly for lower limb supply at this time (McColl, 1986). In 1948, the UK Health Service became a national service (NHS) and the 30 000 civilian amputees now also came under the care of the Ministry of Pensions. The prosthetic company Vessa Ltd was established at this time. Further centres, now known as Artificial Limb and Appliance Centres (ALAC), were opened under the directive of the Ministry of Pensions but they were not always geographically linked to the new hospitals being opened for the NHS at the time.

In 1953, the ALACs in England, Wales and Northern Ireland became the responsibility of the Ministry of Health and 16 new centres were opened, some in the grounds of large general hospitals. In Scotland the service came under the Secretary of State for Scotland and the Limb Fitting Centres became linked to their NHS hospitals. It was not until the late 1960s that Wales and Northern Ireland took over responsibility for their amputees (English and Gregory Dean, 1980). By the late 1950s the greatest number of amputees ever were being cared for by the State, approximately 80 000.

In 1968 the Department of Health and Social Security (DHSS) became responsible for the ALAC services under its Disablement Services Branch. The service continued to be funded by central government and was free of charge to the patient. Patients would have their amputations at an NHS hospital and be referred to the ALAC for prosthetic care under a medical officer. These centres were staffed by DHSS personnel which included medical officers, administrative and clerical staff and, at some centres, nurses, physiotherapists and occupational therapists. The resident medical officer examined the referred patient and prescribed the appropriate limb (DHSS, 1978). The limb or prosthesis is supplied to the DHSS by a limb contractor who manufactures the prosthesis as requested in the prescription. These private companies employ qualified prosthetists (limb fitters) to fit and deliver the limbs. The final acceptance of the limb is dependent upon the medical officer and the patient. In the late 1960s, there were nine artificial limb firms with 1600 employees (BMA, 1968). The DHSS's own technical staff ensured that high standards of manufacture laid down by the department were maintained (DHSS, 1978). The prosthetic companies were paid for the prostheses they supplied at a pre-arranged contractual price. Once the limb had been delivered to the patient, prosthetic training took place at the few ALACs where there was a resident physiotherapist or at the patient's local general hospital. There were 13 basic artificial legs (including pylons) with approximately 100 variations of suspension knee control and feet and 20 basic arms, each in three versions, with a range of terminal devices to cover a variety of occupations and hobbies. By the late 1960s, there were 20 ALACs in England, two in Wales, five in Scotland and one in Northern Ireland and the waiting time for the first limb or pylon was rarely less than 6 weeks (BMA, 1968).

In 1970 the prosthetic services in Scotland were reviewed by the Scottish Home and Health Department (1970), the Denny Report. It recommended that a national centre for training and education in prosthetics and orthotics be set up and that prosthetists and technicians should be employed as in the NHS clinic team. The report also recommended that the service should be seen in the context of a comprehensive rehabilitation service and that the funding, by the Scottish Home and Health Department, should be reviewed. In 1982 a second report was published in Scotland which reviewed not only the prosthetic service but also the orthotic and aids for the disabled service (Hamblen, 1982). Changes in practice followed this report and stimulated the review of such services in the rest of the nation.

The medical officers were generally doctors recruited from the armed forces at the conclusion of their military career. They were employed by the Government through the Ministry of Health rather than through the Health Service and were therefore Civil Servants. They received a 2 month training period at Roehampton and were posted to a provisional centre where supervision and training were continued. In the post First World War days little attempt was made to influence the operating surgeons to produce the best type of stump. It was regarded as the duty of the limb fitting doctors to fit a prosthesis to whatever stump was sent. More recently all ALAC doctors have been expected to integrate fully with the activities of the adjacent hospital and lecture to medical and paramedical staff on amputation surgery and rehabilitation (English and Gregory Dean, 1980). Today medical officers are teaching students and junior surgeons and making them aware of good amputation practice.

The service continued to grow and by 1980 there were ALACs in the towns of Brighton, Bristol, Cambridge, Carlisle, Exeter, Gillingham, Hull, Leeds, Leicester, Liverpool, Harold Wood (Romford, Essex), London (Kingston), London (Balham), London (Ealing), London (Roehampton), Manchester, Middlesborough, Newcastle, Norwich, Nottingham, Oxford, Plymouth, Portsmouth, Preston, Sheffield, Stanmore (Middlesex) and Stoke on Trent (Figure 11.1). Eighteen were main ALACs and nine sub-centres. Thirteen of these centres were in the grounds of a District General Hospital or specialized rehabilitation unit, ten were in the grounds of some other hospital and the remainder were not in hospital grounds.

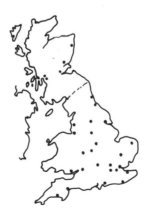

Figure 11.1 Location of Prosthetic Centres in 1984.

THE McCOLL REPORT

In May 1984 a working party was set up 'to review and report on the ιdequacy, quality and management of the various services received by patients in ALACs in England, Wales and Northern Ireland and on the respective roles of the staff of the centres, the NHS and manufacturers, having regard to the need to promote efficiency and cost effectiveness'. The working party consisted of six members and four additional assessors (McColl, 1986). Scotland's limb service has been managed separately for many years.

It was reported that in 1984 these centres dealt with 51 130 lower limb and 11 813 upper limb amputations at a cost of £38 million. Although the ALAC service at this time was responsible for the supply of prostheses, wheelchairs, artificial eyes, surgical appliances for war pensioners and invalid carriages, the medical officers spent the majority of their time dealing with the prosthetic workload. The working party found the problems of the prosthetic centres fell into four main areas: fitting, management, commercial and access.

Fitting

The ill-fitting prostheses were primarily felt to be due to construction mistakes, poorly organized handling of the patients and poorly trained prosthetists. The review, however, also highlighted some other points. In 1972, the British Orthopaedic Association had stated that most amputations were carried out by junior staff who performed few annually. They felt that amputations should be carried out by one surgeon to 'ensure proficiency and some centralisation' and who should be interested in the procedure. Amputating surgeons should have a knowledge of prosthetics and the 'concept of amputation as an operation providing a new organ of locomotion'. The McColl Report highlighted two surveys that showed that 24–37% of all stumps were difficult or impossible to fit with a prosthesis.

McColl recommendations

The report recommended the following:

1. that wherever possible amputations should be carried out in special units where consultant expertise is supported by a multidisciplinary team;

2. that there should be close co-operation between the ALAC medical officer or Clinical Director, the prosthetist and therapist involved with the patient after the surgery;
3. that surgeons should be examined for the diploma of Fellowship of the Royal College of Surgeons, on amputation techniques and post-operative rehabilitation;
4. that low dependency hostel accommodation should be provided near to each ALAC for cost-effective rehabilitation;
5. that each ALAC should have a Clinical Director who is trained in prosthetics, orthotics and rehabilitation and who would be responsible for the full rehabilitation of these disabled people back into the community (it was envisaged that some of the present medical officers would be suitable and some would require further training);
6. that to improve the fitting of prostheses, each patient should be allocated to a prosthetist for continuing service and care or be requested to do so;
7. that a new professional organization should be created to upgrade the present low standards and training of prosthetists; and
8. that therapists must be closely involved with ALAC services wherever they are based. They should be included in the team for proper assessment, prosthetic care, training and general rehabilitation.

Management

The working party found that poor management had produced serious delays and ineffective use of resources. A more integrated system with medical rehabilitation was suggested.

Recommendations

The working party recommended the following:

1. that socket production should be decentralized to local workshops with reappraisal of delivery times;
2. that prosthetists should be monitored for their fitting success rate;
3. that the patient transportation system should be reviewed so that the workload is not concentrated into the hours of 10.30 a.m. to 3.30 p.m.;

4. that the management should become more cost-effective with new general management and new contractural arrangements;
5. that the administrative process, i.e. call-up procedure and patient records, should be altered and modernized by prosthetists making their own appointments and patient records by consolidation and computerization;
6. that amputees should be aware of the prosthetic choices available to them;
7. that complaints about the service from patients should be channelled through the Local Community Health Councils; and
8. that privacy and adequate facilities for children should be made at all centres.

Commercial

Although the limb-making firms sought 'a competitive entrepreneurial spirit that in no way conflicts with the service to the patient' the working party found no real evidence of competition. Each firm's share of the market had not changed significantly over the years and contractors' representation at the centres in the 1970s resulted in the three major firms securing local monopolies. It was also impossible to compare costs per item between one company and another. At centres with more than one contractor, orders tended to be placed on a rota basis. The system was found to reward inefficiency and delay and provided no incentives for suppliers to make improvements for patients, the DHSS and the suppliers themselves. Prosthetists' rates of pay were standardized and therefore there was no poaching of staff between companies. The contractors felt there could be better training programmes for patients in the use of artificial limbs and training to increase the doctors' knowledge of prosthetics. The contractors' opinion of the ALAC medical officers varied from finding them 'helpful and necessary' to being 'totally unnecessary'. The report found that there was a strong disincentive for suppliers to increase their efficiency and reduce costs since it would result in reduced profit levels. Average pricing within a limb group was seen and costs varied by around 890%. Only half of the new limbs and major repairs were delivered on time and a quarter of the general repairs took longer than they should. Professor Radcliffe of Berkeley University, California, said 'Not only do prosthetists in England not know how to apply what is considered to be well recognised principles of modern prosthetic technology, it is often difficult for them to accept criticism from abroad'.

Recommendations

The working party recommended that:

1. the market should be opened up and individual prosthetists encouraged to set up independently;
2. new contracts based on a fee per session should be offered to the present firms and those willing to set up small businesses;
3. contracts should be agreed for the supply of limbs at individually quoted prices and at every centre all types of limbs should be supplied;
4. the suppliers will be responsible for their own products but the management board will have a Technical Director to monitor the results;
5. accounting expertise should be introduced to ensure more effective cost control; and
6. the new management board should be responsible for all research and development (both national and international) and be funded accordingly.

Access

The problem of transportation to the centres and appointments were found by the working party to be unacceptable.

Recommendations

The working party recommended that:

1. amputations should be carried out at a special unit which had access to an ALAC or in which 'fitting could be conducted locally';
2. low dependency hostel accommodation near to the ALAC should be provided;
3. team management of the patients would ensure that each patient would receive the 'walking training required to reach an optimum level' for the individual rather than training continue indefinitely;
4. prosthetists should make their own patient appointments to ensure they give the patients adequate time for fitting;
5. the daily transportation system should be improved to the centres so that the workload covers the whole day (Vessa and Hanger felt they

would be able to provide transport directly and monthly clinics in the remote areas); and
6. domiciliary visits should be considered.

THE DISABLEMENT SERVICES AUTHORITY

Following the publication of the McColl Report in January 1986, a new authority was announced by the Minister for the Disabled on 10 March 1987. This authority, the Disablement Services Authority (DSA) is to run between 1 July 1987 and 31 March 1991 when the service becomes incorporated into the NHS. It is responsible for the following:

1. running the service for the transitional period;
2. building upon the improvements taking place in the service; and
3. overseeing the planning for eventual transfer.

Organization

The Authority is chaired by Lord Holderness (a bilateral amputee) with Professor Lord McColl as the Vice-Chairman and there are eight members. There are 14 Regional Managers with the same boundaries as the Regional Health Authorities.

The Regional Managers are responsible for:

1. all artificial limb and appliance services in their region;
2. their own budgets;
3. managing all medical, administrative and technical staff;
4. planning services;
5. managing and continuing to improve existing services; and
6. planning the integration of these services into existing Health Authorities.

In connection with the artificial limb service, the DSA's aim is to 'bring about an independent prosthetic service capable of fitting a variety of limbs produced by manufacturers in a competitive market, ensuring that each customer's individual needs are met so that the first fitting achieves the desired goals in their total rehabilitation programme'.

Their objectives are:

1. to improve the quality of limb manufacture and fitting and the overall delivery times of limbs and repairs;
2. separate contracts for the supply of artificial limbs and prosthetic services;
3. ensure competition between contractors;
4. secure the improvement of arrangements for prosthetic training; and
5. improve liaison with surgeons to secure better amputation practices (DSA, 1988).

The present (1987–1991)

Each DSA region has a management team comprising of administrative, clinical and technical representations. In principle these are autonomous but in practice there is considerable central input to regional decisions (Luff, 1988). Each DSA region corresponds to its Regional Health Authority and successful liaison is in place with a view to integrating the service into the NHS in 1991. The Regional Managers took control of their budgets in 1989 and financial consultants have installed a financial and internal audit system. The Regional Managers define standards of service for patients in their own regions and continue to monitor the performance of contractors.

In 1989, as a result of competitive tendering, national hardware contracts have provisionally been awarded to 12 firms. For example, LIC, a long established Swedish prosthetic, orthotic and footwear company is now providing prosthetic components and services in Edinburgh, Dundee and Yorkshire and independent companies, such as RSL (Rehabilitation Services Ltd), are practising in the Disablement Service Centres or prosthetic centres. Equipment and accommodation are provided by the State on a leasing scheme. The prosthetic service companies contracted by the DSA are required by contract to offer the full range of hardware, supply the components from the three major modular systems, Endolite, Ultra Roelite and Otto Bock and supply all types of conventional limbs. Some additional training of the prosthetists and technicians in, for example the Otto Bock casting and manufacturing methods, will be necessary before this can be achieved. It is expected that these new contractural arrangements will improve the quality of the service, make the service more flexible, improve the delivery times and make it more cost-effective. With prosthetic publicity, patients are becoming increasingly aware of the prostheses available. The price now paid for the prosthesis is for the limb to be successfully fitted, whereas previous contracts provided little incentive to get it right first time (McColl, 1989). Contractural arrangements for the upper limb supply are now in hand.

Until 1989, the prosthetists were employed by commercial companies which in general limited the freedom of their actions. During 1989, new contractural systems were implemented. These separated the national supply of hardwear from the clinical services provided by the prosthetists. Prosthetists are now encouraged to rectify their own casts locally which should directly contribute to a better fitting prosthesis (McColl, 1989) and an improvement in the professional standing of prosthetists (Luff, 1988). They are also now responsible for making their own patient appointments.

Prosthetists' training had been based in London at The London School of Prosthetics and Paddington College and at the National Centre for Training in Prosthetics and Orthotics, University of Strathclyde, Glasgow. At Paddington College, the course leads to a BTEC Higher National Diploma qualification after 3 years of study and a Diploma awarded by OPTEC (Orthotic and Prosthetic Training and Education Council) after a fourth year of study. At Strathclyde, a 4 year course leads to a BSc in Prosthetics and Orthotics. A shortage in the supply of prosthetists in the UK and the disarray of orthotic training services in England has prompted the DSA to favour a proposal of integrating training of prosthetists and orthotists to degree level in England, probably based at Salford University, and to increase the numbers admitted at Strathclyde University. This will enable the prosthetists training in England, to change from being financially supported by a limb contractor to become independent students as are other health professionals.

In line with the McColl Report, where Clinical Directors were recommended, suitably retrained medical officers are joining the NHS rehabilitation medical teams as Consultant or Clinical Assistants. Multidisciplinary teams both in hospitals and the prosthetic centres are increasing in number and more therapists are being appointed in these centres. In some health regions, low dependency rehabilitation units have been opened (Lumley, 1990, personal communication). Although there has been no official mention of changes in surgical training, international and national meetings are planned for 1990 and 1992 on this topic. Also as recommended in the report, groups have been established to look at various aspects of the prosthetic service, for example medical documentation to revise the system of recording patient information and clinical audit which involves practice and outcome.

Some recommendations have been implemented nationally and some have been and will in the future be only adopted locally.

CONCLUSION

At the beginning of the century, there was no national service for the amputee. Following the First World War a service was set up for the traumatic amputees of the war and gradually the service developed into a national one. However, the client group and management have changed over these years and the service was reviewed in 1986. After a 40 year period of little or no change the last few years have seen complete upheaval for patients and staff alike.

From April 1991, the prosthetic service will be fully integrated into the NHS. The service in each region will have variations to suit the local requirements. The centres that were formerly known as the ALAC, then briefly as the DSC, will probably become known as Prosthetic Centres. Their numbers, locations, staffing and the service they provide, will develop and vary locally. A national (England, Wales and Northern Ireland) prosthetic service will no longer exist but it will be a part of the NHS.

REFERENCES

DHSS (1978) Operation of the British Artificial Limb Service. STB7 Information Service, London.

BMA (1968) Report on the working party on aids for the disabled. Planning Unit Report No.2.

DHSS (1987) Operation of the British Artificial Limb Service, Roehampton.

DSA (1988) *Disablement Services Authority Introductory Guide*. DSA, 13–16 Russell Square, London WC1B 5EP.

English, A.W.G. and Greagory Dean, A.A. (1980) The Artificial Limb Service. *Health Trends*, **12**, 77–82.

Hamblen, D.L. (1982) *Prostheses, Orthoses and Aids for the Disabled*. HMSO, Edinburgh.

Luff, R. (1988) The Artificial Limb Service 1988, in *The Team Approach to the Treatment of Peripheral Vascular Disease, Aetiology to Amputation*, Course Booklet, King's College Hospital School of Medicine and Dentistry, London SE5.

McColl, I. (1986) *Review of the Artificial Limb and Appliance Centre Services*. HMSO, London.

McColl, I. (1989) The Artificial Limb Service is on the move, in *Blesmag*, summer, pp. 6–7.

Scottish Home and Health Department (1970) *The Future of the Artificial Limb Service in Scotland*. HMSO, London.

12

Lower limb prostheses and ambulation

INTRODUCTION

During 1985 there were 5606 lower limb amputees referred to the limb fitting centres in England, Wales and Northern Ireland for prosthetic prescription. The majority of these were for prostheses at the above-knee, transfemoral level (49%) and below-knee, transtibial level (42%) (Ham *et al.*, 1989). Therefore, in the majority of hospital practices, the above- and below-knee amputees are most commonly seen. This chapter will therefore concentrate on these two levels and only discuss briefly amputations at the hip, knee, ankle and foot (Table 12.1).

Until recently, all amputees in the UK received two definitive prostheses. Now the following categories of patients are automatically given two legs: war pensioners, children, people at work, the very active, the overweight, patients who experience stump volume changes and those who are subject to prosthetic breakage. Other patients are given two prostheses only on a medical officer's recommendation. Temporary prostheses are becoming less common as prosthetic supply becomes quicker.

There are currently two types of prosthetic system available today: exoskeletal and endoskeletal. The exoskeletal system requires a greater number of man hours for construction and alterations to the alignment or socket. It is, however, more robust and preferred by the active, heavier patient. The endoskeletal or modular system reduces the assembly costs of the prosthesis and the components are easily adjusted and exchanged. The system has a soft foam cosmesis with a prosthetic skin cover or stocking. (British prosthetic codes and abbreviations are given in Appendix 12.1.)

The lower limb of the body accounts for 18.6% of a person's total

Table 12.1 Major levels of lower limb amputation (DHSS, England, Wales and Northern Ireland, 1985)

Through hip	0.5%
Above knee	49%
Through knee	4%
Below knee	42%
Around the foot	1%

body weight. This is important to remember when noting the weight of the lower limb prosthesis and patients' comments regarding this.

ABOVE-KNEE (TRANSFEMORAL) PROSTHESES

The above-knee prosthesis has six main component parts: the suspension, the socket, the knee joint and knee control mechanisms, the shank and the ankle and foot device (Figure 12.1a, b).

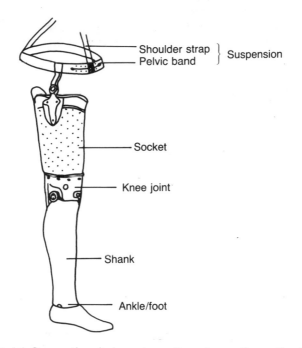

Figure 12.1 (a) Conventional above-knee (transfemoral) prosthesis.

Fig 2. 171

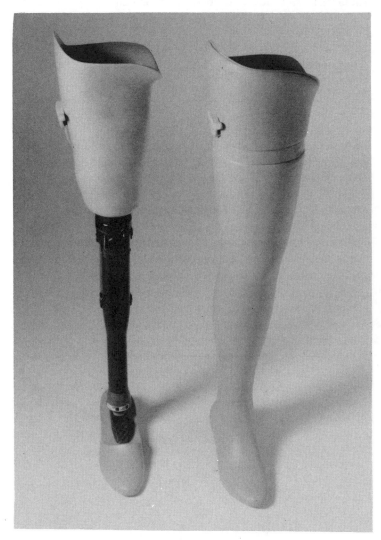

Figure 12.1 (b) Endolite above-knee modular prosthesis.

Suspension

There are six types of suspension commonly used: the pelvic band, silesian bandage or belt, total elastic suspension (TES) belt, the suction socket, the total surface bearing socket and the shoulder strap.

Pelvic band

The pelvic band is made up of a metal (usually aluminium) 'T'-shaped bar which is attached to the socket inferiorly and covered with leather at the pelvis forming a belt. The metal 'T' bar also incorporates a hip joint. This can either be uniaxial, allowing only flexion and extension to take place (the rigid pelvic band, RPB) or multiaxial, either semi-double switch allowing flexion, extension and rotation or double-switch allowing flexion, extension, rotation, abduction and adduction to take place (the double swivel pelvic band, DSPB) (Figure 12.2). The band should be situated between the iliac crests and the greater trochanters on the pelvis. It provides not only suspension to the above-knee prosthesis but also helps to control rotation which gives a more rigid gait. It does, however, add 0.5–1.5 kg to the weight of the prosthesis and is uncomfortable for the amputee when sitting (Sanders, 1986b). It can be

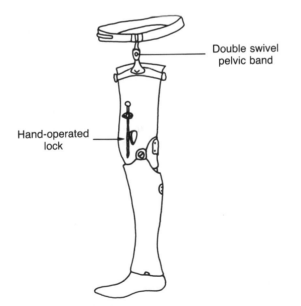

Double swivel
pelvic band

Hand-operated
lock

Figure 12.2 Above-knee prosthesis with DSPB.

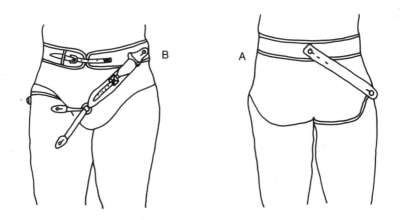

Figure 12.3 Silesian belt.

noisy and tear or stain clothing, although leather clothes guards are available. It is beneficial with the short stump where suction is impossible.

Silesian belt

The silesian belt is a non-elastic webbing that is attached to the lateral wall of the prosthesis and passes posteriorly around the pelvis between the iliac crest and greater trochanter and attaches to the socket anteriorly at the height of the ischial tuberosity (Figure 12.3). Stud A should be placed at the centre back and stud B at the iliac crest. The back strap attaches to the posterolateral stud of the socket preventing medial rotation of the prosthesis. The front strap attaches to two studs on the anterior aspect of the socket and prevent lateral rotation. Buckles fasten the belt and front strap. The attachment was originally bifurcated but is often now seen as a single attachment and uses an adjustable buckle or velcro. The silesian belt is lighter and more comfortable than the pelvic band and does not resist hip mobility. It is often used as an auxiliary to a suction socket, especially during the early stages of suction use.

Total elastic suspension belt

The TES belt comes in three sizes, small, medium and large, and the size required is taken from the socket circumference. It is made of

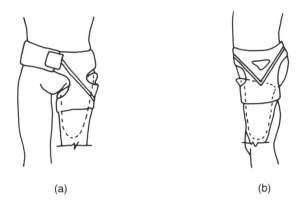

(a)   (b)

Figure 12.4 TES belt. (a) Front view (b) lateral view.

neoprene, closes anteriorly with velcro and is washable. The TES belt is pulled onto the socket and then pulled up onto the pelvis when donning is complete (Figure 12.4).

Suction socket – self-suspension

Although there are records of suction sockets in 1863 it was not until after the Second World War that such sockets were popularized (Sanders, 1986a). A one-way valve is fitted on the medial and inferior aspect of the socket. The amputee wears either a sock or a bandage on his stump which he then threads out through the valve hole, pulling down the stump tissue into the socket. The valve is pushed into position and as the amputee bears weight, the remaining air is expelled through the one-way valve, creating a negative pressure or suction effect. It is essential that the stump socket fit is accurate for this negative pressure to be maintained.

The suction method is contraindicated with vascular problems and where there are fluctuations in the size of the stump or where there are alterations in body weight. Psychological or emotional difficulties in some patients can also be contraindications for its choice (Sanders, 1986a). It is also difficult to achieve suspension on a short stump. The advantages of the suction socket are that it is cosmetically more acceptable and more comfortable. The disadvantages are that it causes suction oedema, requires an intimate fit and increases sweating and possible skin problems. It is sometimes found to be noisy when suction is reduced and it requires a mature stump without fluctuating volume. A suction socket is not suitable for the elderly or those with vascular disease who are unable to bend down for a long time to apply the socket. The suction socket is chiefly used for young, fit amputees with stumps that are medium to long in length, as the muscle tension created on walking helps to hold the socket in position.

Total surface bearing socket

Total surface bearing (TSB) or total contact sockets are becoming increasingly popular. In previous socket designs, socket forces were distributed so that more weight was taken by tissues that are thought to be pressure tolerant and forces relieved over tissues that are pressure sensitive. In a TSB socket, weight is distributed more or less evenly over the entire residual surface (Staats and Lundir, 1987).

Shoulder harness and straps

The shoulder harness was used in the past to suspend conventional sockets. With the quadrilateral design of socket, the shoulder harness is almost obsolete and is used only with long-standing cases or as a last resort (Sanders, 1986b). It was replaced by pelvic band suspension in the 1940s (Sanders, 1986a). Shoulder straps are, however, used with elderly patients to assist suspension with a pelvic band (Figure 12.1).

The socket

The most commonly seen shape of above-knee socket today is the quadrilateral socket. Other designs include the conventional, 'H' (Health), the flexible and ischial containment sockets. The sockets are either individually made or modular components and the materials commonly used are metal and plastics. Three centres are currently collaborating to produce a shaping, sensing, computer-aided, socket design system to replace the procedure of hand crafting and modified stump model.

Quadrilateral socket

This socket was designed in the 1950s to accommodate the myoplastic stump. The socket has anterior, posterior, medial and lateral walls (Figure 12.5). The anterior and posterior walls accommodate flexion and extension stump forces during gait and the medial and lateral walls

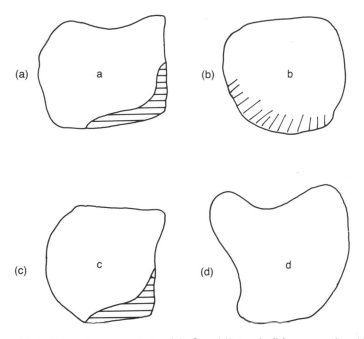

Figure 12.5 Above-knee sockets. (a) Quadrilateral, (b) conventional/plug, (c) 'H' (Health), (d) ischial containment.

provide stability in the stance phase. The anterior and lateral walls are 5 cm higher and the posterior wall incorporates an ischial shelf for a weight-bearing surface for the ischium. The extra height of the anterior wall ensures that the ischium remains on the shelf or platform. This design of socket provides better pressure distribution for the stump and promotes venous return (Sanders, 1986a). The quadrilateral socket is criticized for being a non-anatomical shape and providing poor stump control in the coronal plane. The ischial seating on this prosthesis and the alignment over the prosthetic foot cannot simulate a feeling of weight bearing through the hip joint (Flandry *et al.*, 1989).

Conventional (plug fit or trumpet) socket

This type of socket was used between 1914 and the late 1940s and its shape accommodates the conical non-myoplastic stump of the period. Problems with swelling, ulceration at the end of the stump and proximal skin rolls were seen with this type of socket (English and Dean, 1980), weight bearing was through the active socket (Figure 12.5).

'H' (Health) socket

In 1949 at Roehampton, McKenzie developed the 'H' socket, a triangular-shaped socket which incorporated for the first time an ischial platform (Figure 12.5). It was commonly used in the UK until the 1980s.

Ischial containment sockets

Ischial containment sockets were developed in the late 1980s by three centres in the USA (Figure 12.5). The major difference in this socket's design compared with the quadrilateral socket is that the ischial tuberosity is contained within the socket, altering the socket brim and the medial and lateral diameters have been reduced, making the shape oval in an anterior and posterior direction. The socket provides more room for the stump to move in flexion and extension and therefore functions more naturally (Mensch and Ellis, 1987). From the University of California at Los Angeles (UCLA) the contoured adducted trochanteric/controlled alignment method (CAT/CAM) has been developed, chiefly by Sabolich. At the North Western University at Chicago, the normal shape normal alignment (NSNA) design has been developed

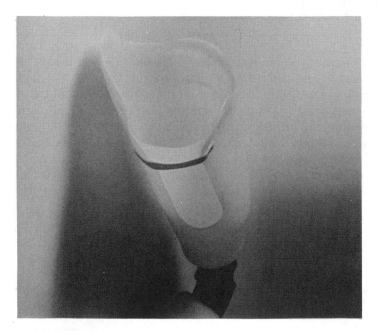

Figure 12.6 (a) Ischial containment socket.

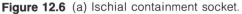

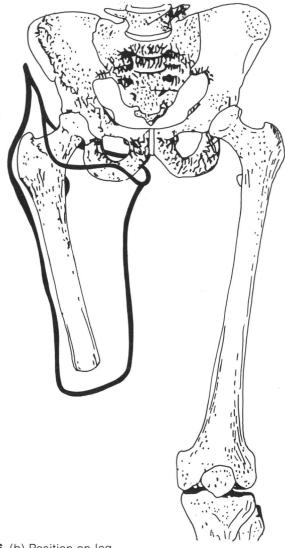

Figure 12.6 (b) Position on leg.

and at New York University the narrow medio lateral (Narrow ML)
design (Figure 12.6a, b).

The wrap cast of the stump is taken with the patient standing and
currently it is being used for younger athletic patients. Several check
sockets are used to obtain the correct fit. Patients subjectively rate this
socket favourably. The mean stride length and gait velocity improved

179

and the oxygen consumption decreased using this socket compared with a quadrilateral socket. It increased the patient's socket comfort, stability and balance and only a short period of time was required in the conversion from a quadrilateral socket (Flandry *et al.*, 1989).

ISNY flexible socket

The ISNY (Iceland, Sweden, New York) socket was introduced in 1984 following development that was started by an Icelandic prosthetist, Ossur Kristinsson, Een Holmgren in Sweden and then included the New York Postgraduate Medical School. The design challenged the previous hard socket principles. The socket consists of two structures, the hard socket and the soft flexible socket. The hard socket has two functions, weight bearing and stump accommodation. The flexible socket has two components, the socket which is a vacuum-formed quadrilateral socket made of transparent polyethylene, providing total contact and the carbon fibre support frame which provides stability and transmits weight-bearing forces (Figure 12.7). Derivations of this design are also seen in the UK.

The advantages of this socket are that it is light and provides greater comfort and increased sensation and proprioception. It is more pliable when sitting and it dissipates heat faster than traditional sockets (Mensch, 1984). The ISNY socket has been used with the fitter adult amputee and children from the age of 5 years.

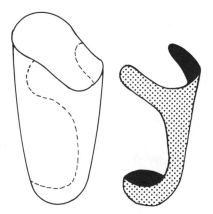

Figure 12.7 ISNY above-knee flexible socket illustrating the rigid frame (right) and its final position on the socket.

Knee joints

Knee joints function like hinges and are activated by stump movements. They must flex easily and provide stability under load. Some knee joints increase stance stability whereas others enhance the gait pattern by assisting the swing phase (Radcliffe, 1977). They are divided into two groups: single axis and polycentric joints.

Single or uniaxis

The rotation centre of the joint is fixed in one point in all the knee positions (Öberg and Kamwendo, 1988). Extension is maintained by hip extension and the prosthetic contact with the ground (Mensch and Ellis, 1987).

Polycentric axis

The rotation centre has different locations in different angular positions of the knee, i.e. there are many joint centres (Öberg and Kamwendo, 1988). Polycentric knees attempt to duplicate the function of the anatomical knee to provide increased knee stability. Different systems use different designs, for example the polycentric two and four bar linkage knees. With the four bar linkage joint for example, the polygon position of the bars projects the centre of rotation proximally and posteriorly to give stance stability (Fernie and Ruder, 1981a) and assists in shortening the prosthetic shank during the swing phase by moving the centre of rotation anteriorly and distally (Radcliffe, 1977). It is therefore especially useful for the amputee with a knee disarticulation.

Knee control mechanisms

Knee control mechanisms can be divided into stance phase controls and swing phase controls.

Stance phase controls

Stance phase controls are required for those amputees who require knee stability at the beginning of the stance phase and when walking on rough ground (Fernie and Ruder, 1981a; Mensch and Ellis, 1987). They

181

provide a safer, more confident gait and stance phase stability is achieved by alignment or by a variety of locking mechanisms (Sanders, 1986b). An example is the Endolite stabilized knee. The Endolite stance flex knee allows some flexion at mid-stance, hence shortening the prosthesis without releasing the weight-activated knee stabilizer and therefore reducing energy expenditure as the amputee does not have to rise over the prosthesis at mid-stance.

Swing phase controls

Swing phase control mechanisms work in a similar way to car shock absorbers or the damping units fitted to stop doors slamming (Fernie and Ruder, 1981a). Their function is to control the forward motion of the shank during swing phase and reducing heel rise. Various designs are available which include function, pneumatic and hydraulic dampers, and external and internal extension bias systems (Sanders, 1986b). The pneumatic swing phase control unit is an example and Blatchford's is the most commonly used in the UK.

The shank or calf

The shank (Figure 12.1) was traditionally exoskeletal in its design and made of metal. Today endoskeletal, modular systems made up of a metal rod with a soft cover are more common.

Ankle foot devices

There are five ankle and foot devices commonly used today.

Uniaxial or single axis ankle foot

This conventional foot allows 5°–7° of dorsiflexion and 15° plantarflexion. It is a hinge joint that is restricted in movement by two rubber bumpers, the plantarflexion and dorsiflexion bumpers (Figure 12.8). The advantages of this type of device is that it has a range of movement that is adjustable, it is economical and easy to maintain and it allows the foot to be placed flat without much force on the heel ensuring knee stability (Sanders, 1986d). Its disadvantage is that the rubber parts wear and become noisy, it is heavy, cosmetically poor and allows no

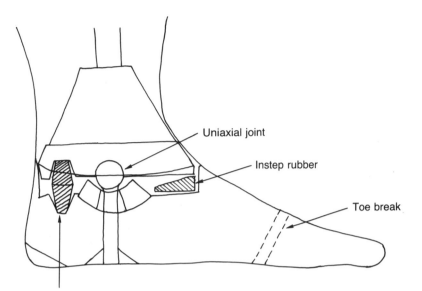

Figure 12.8 Single axis foot.

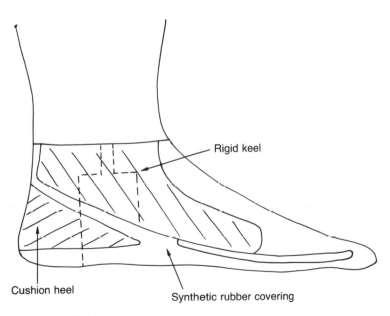

Figure 12.9 SACH foot.

rotation at the ankle and foot joints. Until recently this type of foot was commonly seen in the UK either made of wood or plastic.

Solid ankle cushion heel foot

The solid ankle cushion heel (SACH) foot was developed in the mid 1950s by Foort and Radcliffe in the USA (Figure 12.9). The foot and ankle are combined into one unit and therefore no articulated ankle joint is required. Movement is provided by the materials used, the soft rubber heel compressing under load (Sanders, 1986c). Three varieties of density are available, soft, medium and hard. Its advantages are that there are no moving parts and therefore maintenance is low, it has a better cosmetic appearance than the uniaxial foot, it is light and provides a smooth heel strike toe off movement. It is generally prescribed for children as it stands up to wear and tear. Its disadvantages are that the material used gradually loses its elasticity and the amount of dorsi- and plantarflexion possible is limited.

Multiaxis ankle and foot device

The multiaxis device allows some movement in all three planes of movement at the ankle. It was generally used for the more active amputee but is now standard issue in the UK. The Blatchfords Multiflex is an example (Figure 12.10).

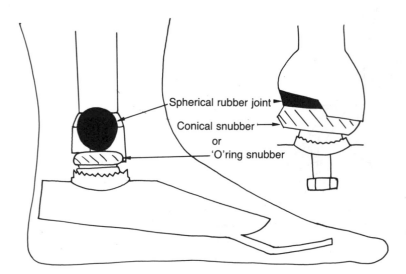

Spherical rubber joint

Conical snubber
or
'O'ring snubber

Figure 12.10 Multiflex foot. (a) Joint within limb.

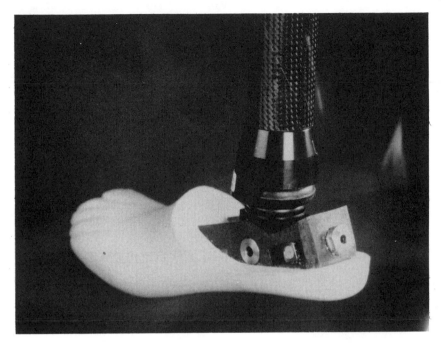

Figure 12.10 (b) Exposed ankle joint.

Seattle foot

The Seattle foot was developed in the early 1980s by the Prosthetic Research Study of the University of Washington in Seattle. The foot can be 'lifelike', the lifecast model or a traditional shape, the smoothie model. Both incorporate an energy-storing Delrin heel which is released at a rate compatible with each forward movement of the patient to produce a natural lift and thrust to the foot. When using the Seattle foot walking and running are more effective and less tiring (Beswick, 1986). A separate large toe and the natural foot appearance make it possible to wear sandals. The Seattle foot is, however, heavy (Figure 12.11).

Quantum foot

The Vessa Quantum foot is the first device to simulate flexion between the heel and toe and lateral movement at the ankle joint (Figure 12.12). It is composed of two heels made of glass fibre in epoxy resin. The upper

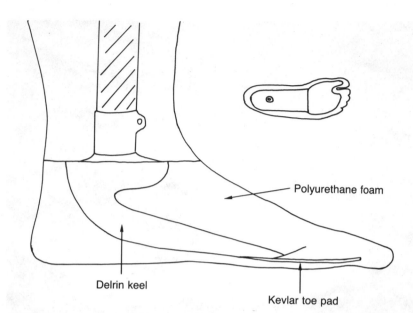

Figure 12.11 Seattle foot.

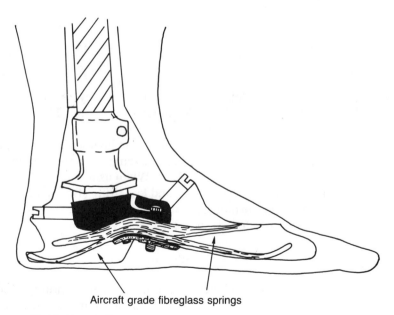

Aircraft grade fibreglass springs

Figure 12.12 Vessa Quantum foot.

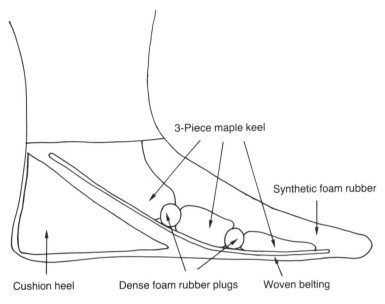

Figure 12.13 Sten foot.

member provides rigidity and the lower one, which is longer and thinner, provides the spring in the step by flexing the toe and heel portions of the prosthesis. The foot comes in different weights, spring rates and different foot sizes. The foot is hollow, which allows it to fit more easily into shoes. A heel height adjuster is planned for the future.

Other examples

Other variations of feet can also be seen (Edelstein, 1988). For example, the energy stored STEN foot (Figure 12.13), the SAFE (Stationery attachment flexible endoskeleton) foot (Figure 12.14) which is a modified SACH foot, the Flex foot (Figure 12.15) and the Jaipur foot, which was originally designed by Dr P. K. Sethi for Indian beggars and allows the amputee to walk barefoot, work in the fields and sit cross legged on the floor. The Jaipur foot is made from vulcanized rubber with a layer of nylon cord inside (similar to car tyres).

In the UK approximately 85% of amputees, until recently, were fitted with uniaxial feet, whereas in the USA 80% use the SACH foot. In a recent study the uniaxial foot was found more closely to resemble the normal foot in providing plantarflexion in early stance. The SACH foot

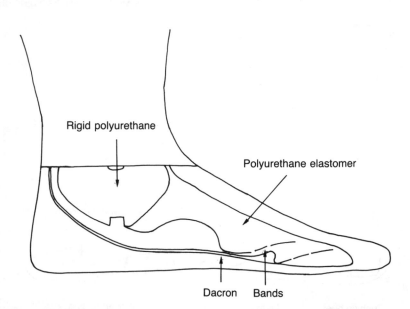

Figure 12.14 SAFE foot.

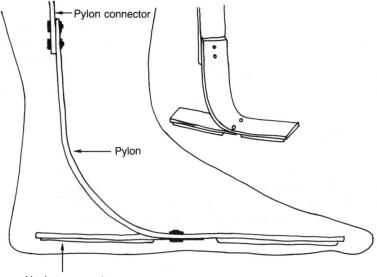

Figure 12.15 Flex foot.

gave a smoother transition from heel strike to toe off. With proper selection of heel stiffness and prosthetic alignment similar results can be achieved. If cost is also considered the SACH would be the first choice for the unilateral active below- and above-knee amputee (Goh *et al.*, 1984). Less active amputees may benefit from the uniaxial foot which brings the foot into contact with the ground early, so providing better support and stability. The newer designs, for example the Quantum, are yet to be evaluated but are becoming more widely available in the UK.

Rehabilitation points

Application or donning

Prior to donning check that:

1. the prosthesis is the correct one for the patient;
2. the hip, knee and ankle mechanisms are understood and are working smoothly;
3. the socket has no sharp edges and has a smoothly finished interior;
4. any leatherwork is firmly attached;
5. the patient's shoe fits the foot properly and is not excessively worn; and
6. his shoes are a pair and that the shoe for the prosthesis is the original shoe given to the prosthetist, or exactly the same heel height (Barsby, 1989, personal communication).

Standard socket

The above-knee prosthesis is generally applied in the sitting position. The sock is first applied well up the stump and the pelvic band is placed anterior to the socket. The prosthesis is applied flexed with the toe slightly rotated laterally and once the socket contains the stump the pelvic band is located and fastened. The sock is pulled up over the socket and finally the shoulder strap is located and fixed. The patient then puts on his pants and dresses himself normally.

Suction socket

Talcum powder is generally applied to the stump to reduce the friction of application. In sitting, a sock or bandage with a lace or pulling string attached distally is applied to the stump. All the proximal soft tissue is included in this bandage. The prosthetic valve is removed and the covered limb inserted into the socket. The pulling string, lace or loose edge of bandage is threaded through the valve hole and then the patient stands to continue pulling the stump into position. Soft tissue must be palpable or visible through the valve hole for the application to have been successful. With the patient's full weight on the prosthesis the valve is replaced. When the amputee starts to walk there should be no noise heard of air escaping. If there is noise or if soft tissue is not palpated through the valve hole, the prosthesis must be reapplied.

Static check out

Following donning the following anatomical areas should be checked in the prosthesis.

1. The ischial tuberosity should rest on the posterior shelf of the socket. The patient should be asked to take his weight off the prosthesis initially, the therapist should locate the ischial tuberosity and then ask the patient to bear weight.
2. The adductor longus tendon should lie in the medial corner of the socket, medial to Scarpa's bulge if it has been built into the socket. It should be palpated by the therapist and the patient then asked to contract his adductor muscles against resistance. The tendon should be felt in the adductor groove of the socket.
3. The greater trochanter should be located in the middle of the lateral side of the socket (Picken, 1985).
4. The medial soft tissues should be contained in the socket and not lie above it producing an adductor roll.
5. In standing the length of the prosthesis should be checked by palpating the iliac crests and the anterior superior iliac spines. Temporary prostheses are often made 1–2 cm shorter to assist the patient in the swing phase of initial gait training. The position of the pelvic band and the shoulder strap if used should be checked. The strap must be adjusted to allow a flat hand to be passed between the patient's skin and the strap. If the strap is too tight the patient will stoop forward and if it is too loose the suspension of the limb will be inadequate.

Use

During the training period, the patient will be encouraged to increase gradually the amount of time he wears his prosthesis, once the initial problems, if any, have been resolved. The patient's skin condition, suture line, skin colour and oedema will need to be regularly observed and recorded.

Dynamic check out

The amputee should be observed from the front and back and from the side. The most common gait deviations are:

1. lateral bending of the trunk;*
2. abducted gait;*
3. circumducted gait;*
4. vaulting;*
5. rotation of the foot on heel strike;
6. uneven arm swing;
7. uneven timing;*
8. uneven heel rise;
9. instability of prosthetic knee;*
10. swing phase whips;
11. foot slap;
12. drop off;
13. uneven length of steps;* and
14. lumbar lordosis* (Karacoloff, 1985).

(The gait deviations marked *are discussed later in this chapter.)

Common problems

If excessive pressure is felt on the residual limb it is lying too low in the socket and the patient will generally complain of pain on his pubic symphysis and medial aspects of the socket. If the tuberosity slides down inside the socket, the socket may be too large, or the stump may have shrunk. This is common with primary amputees and extra stump socks can be worn to compensate. If the tuberosity is above the seating, the socket may be too small (stump plugged out of socket) or oedema is present. A thinner stump sock can be worn or stump volume reduced by bandaging, stump shrinker or using Ppam Aid prior to donning of the prosthesis. If a leather adjustable socket has been prescribed, the socket can be adjusted by the physiotherapist.

Gait training

The following movements should be practised with the new above-knee prosthesis in parallel bars:

1. sitting to standing;
2. balancing on the prosthesis;
3. lateral weight transference;
4. anterior and posterior weight transference;
5. hip hitching;
6. steps taken forward and laterally for stance phase control;
7. swing the prosthesis forward and place the foot to practise swing phase control;
8. stepping forward with the good leg; and
9. walking in the parallel bars ensuring the patient has an upright posture, even stride length and timing and is bearing full weight on the prosthesis.

The exercises should continue using perhaps one stick and one bar and then two sticks. Once the patient's gait is reasonable and his balance good the exercises are continued out of the parallel bars in the gym area. For those patients who are suitable, the programme must continue with practice functionally on stairs, inclines, getting up from the floor, falling, picking up objects, outside surfaces and, for example, public transport. Before discharge, the patient must be able to don and doff his prosthesis and have a knowledge of his sock supply and their use during periods of shrinkage and swelling, care of his prosthesis and his stump.

Common gait deviations

Alignment is discussed on page 215 of this chapter.

Lateral bending of the trunk

Causes:

1. short prosthesis;
2. insufficient support by lateral wall of socket;
3. abducted socket;

4. pain or discomfort on a particular aspect of stump;
5. weak abductors; and
6. walking with abducted gait.

Abducted gait

Large width of walking base. Causes:

1. prosthesis too long;
2. shank aligned in valgus position with respect to thigh section;
3. contracted abductors of stump;
4. feeling of insecurity or fear, patient compensates with wide walking base;
5. pain or discomfort in crotch area; and
6. prosthetic hip joint set so that the socket and stump are abducted.

Circumduction

Lateral curve as prosthesis swings through. Causes:

1. prosthesis too long;
2. manual knee lock preventing knee bending;
3. inadequate suspension allowing prosthesis to slip off stump;   ⎱ Add to
4. socket too small;   ⎰ problem of excessive length
5. foot set in plantar flexion; and
6. insecurity – little or no knee flexion.

Vaulting

Bobbing up and down, by excessively plantar flexing sound foot. Causes:

1. prosthesis too long;
2. inadequate suspension allowing prosthesis to slip off;   ⎱ Add to
3. excessive friction of prosthetic knee of manual knee lock;   ⎰ problem of excessive length
4. socket too small;
5. foot set in plantar flexion; and
6. fear and insecurity.

Uneven timing

Steps of unequal duration, usually a short stance phase on prosthetic side. Causes:

1. improperly fitting socket may cause pain, and therefore patient shortens stance phase on prosthetic side;
2. weak extensor aid or insufficient friction in prosthetic knee, causing excessive heel rise and therefore results in uneven timing because of prolonged swing through;
3. alignment stability if knee buckles too easily;
4. weak stump;
5. poor balance; and
6. fear and insecurity.

Instability of prosthetic knee

Tendency to buckle during prosthetic stance phase, creating a danger of falling. Causes:

1. the knee joint may be too far ahead of the trochanter, knee and ankle line;
2. insufficient initial flexion may have been built into the socket;
3. plantar flexion resistance may be too great causing the knee to buckle at heel strike;
4. failure to limit dorsiflexion can lead to incomplete knee control;
5. weak hip extensors; and
6. severe hip flexion contractures may cause instability.

Uneven length of steps

Length of steps with prosthesis differ from length of steps taken with sound foot, i.e. usually longer. Causes:

1. pain or fear will cause the amputee to get his weight off the prosthesis and onto his sound leg as quickly as possible;
2. therefore he takes short steps with his sound foot;
3. insufficient friction on the prosthetic knee, causing a pendulum-type swing of shank; and
4. flexion contracture of hip or insufficient flexion of socket.

Lumbar lordosis

Normal convexity of lumbar area is exaggerated when prosthesis is in stance phase. Causes:

1. flexion contracture of hip;
2. insufficient initial flexion of socket;
3. insufficient support from brim of anterior socket wall;
4. weak extensors of hip;
5. weak abdominal muscles; and
6. painful ischial bearing (University of Strathclyde, 1980a).

BELOW-KNEE (TRANSTIBIAL) PROSTHESES

The below-knee prosthesis has four main parts: the suspension, socket, shank and ankle and foot mechanism. The shank and ankle and foot devices have been described for the above-knee prosthesis. The below-knee suspension and sockets will be described here.

Suspension

The two most commonly used types of suspension for the below-knee prosthesis are the thigh corset of the conventional limb and the cuff suspension strap or supracondylar cuff of the patella tendon bearing socket (PTB).

Thigh corset

The thigh corset which is made of leather was most commonly used with the earlier type of plug fit socket. It consists of metal sidebars, which incorporate a joint at the knee and attaches to the socket and the shank (Figure 12.16). The thigh corset supports part of the body weight in stance, increasing mediolateral stability of the knee and is therefore helpful where there is muscle weakness or a short stump. As the prosthetic knee joint is a simple single axis joint and the human knee is not, some movement takes place between the limb and the prosthesis with a possibility of chafing. The thigh corset is bulky, cosmetically poor, can cause muscle atrophy if used for a long time and the leather does gradually deform under load. However, amputees who carry out

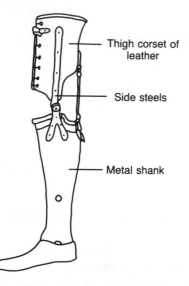

Thigh corset of
leather

Side steels

Metal shank

Figure 12.16 Conventional below-knee prosthesis.

Fig3

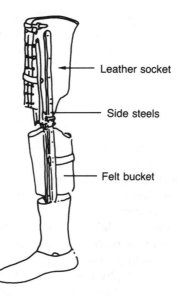

Leather socket

Side steels

Felt bucket

Figure 12.17 Above-knee/below-knee prosthesis: for below-knee amputee requiring a thigh corset.

heavy physical work find this type of suspension to be more supportive. In the UK it is coded No.8. When a below-knee stump is swollen or slow to heal an above-knee/below-knee prosthesis may be prescribed. This is ischial weight bearing with an adjustable thigh corset, semi-automatic knee lock and a felt bucket or cup (Figure 12.17a, b). A rigid pelvic belt may be provided for extra control.

Supracondylar or suprapatella cuff

The leather cuff attaches by studs to the proximal part of the socket in a posteromedial and posterolateral position (Figure 12.18). The cuff circumducts the thigh above the femoral condyles and patella and is closed with either a buckle D ring or velcro laterally. The cuff holds the prosthesis in place during the swing phase and stops hyperextension in stance. In some cases a second strap is added, a 'pick up strap', which is attached around the patient's waist to assist in swing. This type of suspension allows normal movements to take place at the knee and is light and easy to apply. However, it does not give any mediolateral stability and the positioning of the studs is critical (Sanders, 1986d). An elastic insert is occasionally added to improve the fit over the proximal patella border but this is not liked by some as it does not aid in preventing hyperextension.

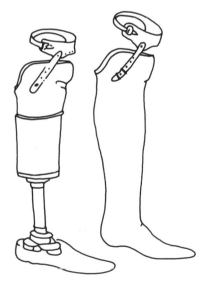

Figure 12.18 PTB prosthesis with supracondylar cuff.

Variations

The other types of suspension seen with below-knee prostheses are the inverted 'Y' strap or fork strap which is attached to a waist band, a neoprene rubber sleeve which covers the knee and the lower third of the thigh, a thick elasticated full length stocking attached to a corset or suspender belt for ladies and suction suspension (currently used in Sweden). Two types of socket incorporate suspension in their design. They will be discussed in the next section.

The socket

All below-knee prostheses have an inner and outer socket. The inner socket is commonly called the liner and the outer socket the shell. The liner is commonly made from pelite, though other materials are becoming available, for example the PI Medical Ice Ross.

Conventional below-knee socket

The traditional below-knee socket which was used with the thigh corset was plug shaped, similar to the early above-knee socket (Figure 12.11).

Patella tendon bearing socket

In 1959 at the University of California the PTB socket was introduced (Figure 12.18). The design provides a more intimate fit and more efficient distribution of pressure around the stump than the No.8 prosthesis. It is a total contact socket, though not endbearing, which increases the weight-bearing capacity of the stump, helps to control oedema and increase proprioception (Mensch and Ellis, 1987). It is shaped like a triangle and the medial and lateral walls are higher than the anterior and posterior. The posterior wall has a flare in it to accommodate knee flexion and make the socket more comfortable in the sitting position. There are also grooves for the hamstrings and gastrocnemius tendons and the posterior wall is concave so that the soft tissues below the popliteal fossa are pushed anteriorly to enforce weight bearing on the formed patella tendon bar. The socket is held in some flexion (approximately 9°) and knee flexion of up to 15° can be generally accommodated with this socket. Relief is given to the crest of the tibia, tibial tubercle, fibula head and cut ends of the fibula and tibia, the patella and when necessary, the prominent lateral tibial condyle, by loading pressure-tolerant areas (Figure 12.19). The pressure- or

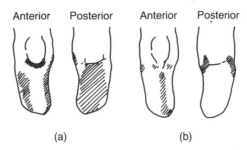

Figure 12.19 Below-knee stump. (a) Pressure-tolerant and (b) pressure-sensitive areas.

weight-tolerant areas are chiefly the patella tendon, medial tibial, the pretibial muscles and the posterior aspect of the stump. When worn correctly the patella sits half in and half out of the prosthesis.

Suction sockets are available for below-knee prostheses but a recent survey in the USA showed that only 22% of prosthetists had made this type of prosthesis (Roberts, 1986). An insert or liner is used with total contact sockets to provide additional cushioning and protect the remaining limb from abrasions during ambulation. They are made from a variety of materials that include pelite, kemble and leather, and silicone gel.

Prosthese tibiale supracondylienne socket

The prosthese tibiale supracondylienne (PTS) below-knee socket was designed by Fajal of France in 1963. It differs from the PTB socket in that the mediolateral brims extend proximally and the socket walls finish above the femoral condyles and enclose the whole of the patella. The patella bar is less pronounced. Often a wedge is placed between the stump and the socket above the medial femoral condyle to provide a close fit and suspension. The PTS restricts movement less than the PTB worn with a cuff and provides greater medial lateral stability. However, it is heavier than a PTB prosthesis and is difficult to use with long below-knee stumps. It also tends to slip down when the knee is flexed to 90° and the leg is off the ground (Sanders, 1986e).

Kondyler bettung Münster socket

The Kondyler bettung Münster (KBM) socket was developed in Münster, Germany, in the early 1960s. It differs from the PTB in that it has higher medial and lateral brims, but unlike the PTS it exposes the

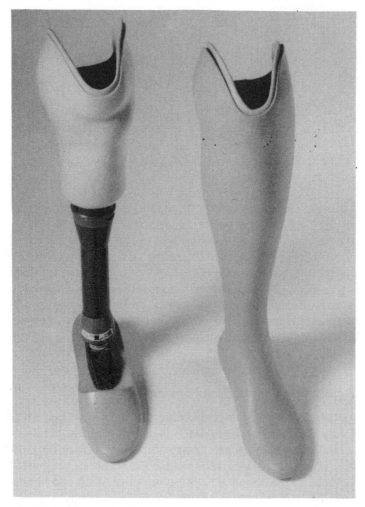

Figure 12.20 KBM prosthesis.

patella (Figure 12.20). This design provides more medial and lateral stability than a PTB and better suspension, especially for the shorter stump. At 90° flexion the suspension is better than with the PTS but its construction and the position of the wedge are crucial for its performance.

Total surface bearing sockets

Sockets that distribute the weight more or less equally over the entire residual limb surface are becoming increasingly popular (Staats, 1989).

The shank and ankle/foot devices are discussed earlier in the Above-knee prostheses section.

Rehabilitation points

Donning

Prior to donning, examine the prosthesis and make sure that:

1. it is the correct one for the patient;
2. his shoes are a pair and the original ones given to the prosthetist;
3. the limb stands upright in the shoe and the foot is flat on the floor; and
4. the knee is in neutral, neither flexed nor extended.

With the patient sitting, one woollen stump sock is donned. (Often a nylon sock is added first to reduce friction between skin and socket.) The soft white pelite liner (or similar) should be eased firmly over the stump and stump sock and the patella tendon bar should rest on the tendon. With some liners socks are not used, for example the Ice Ross. The outer hard socket should then be applied over the liner and when pressure is applied to the prosthesis, it should not slip further onto the stump. The suprapatellar cuff can then be firmly fastened, but enough space should be left to allow two fingers to pass underneath it, preventing a tourniquet effect developing (Barsby, 1989, personal communication).

Static check out

By donning the liner only, the stump can be palpated to check that the weight-tolerant areas are in contact with the socket. This is chiefly the patella tendon bar which should rest over the patella tendon. Weight-tolerant areas also include the muscles on the medial tibial aspect, the anterior tibial compartment, and the posterior distal portion of the stump. These should also be checked after walking a short distance to see if sock marks will appear over these areas. In sitting the contact area between the hamstrings and the socket should be checked to ensure there is enough allowance for the patient to sit with his foot on the floor. In standing, the leg length should be checked by palpating the iliac crests and the anterior or posterior superior iliac spines. The cuff and side straps should be firm enough to maintain suspension and the prosthetic foot should be in contact with the floor. The knee generally should be held in the neutral position, not held in flexion or extension.

Use

It is important that with a new below-knee total contact socket the patient wears the prosthesis for short periods of time initially and that the stump is continually checked for areas of friction. The length of time it is worn will gradually increase as rehabilitation progresses. During this time extra socks will be necessary as the new or primary patient's stump shrinks over a 3–6 month period. Before discharge from physiotherapy the patient must be able to don and doff the prosthesis unaided and understand the variety, use and care of the prosthetic socks. Patients with above-knee/below-knee prostheses should be taught how to don and doff the limb, fasten the leather socket evenly and not too tightly at the proximal or distal ends. They should also be taught how to unlock and lock their limb and check their leg position in the limb with reference to the patella and felt bucket. The patient should be reminded that the prosthesis has been set up for one particular heel height and this should not be altered without discussing it with the prosthetist.

Dynamic check out

The amputee should be observed both from the front and the back and the side. The most common gait deviations are:

1. excessive knee extension or flexion at heel strike;
2. knee extension between mid stance and toe off; and
3. drop off between heel rise and toe off.

The amputee should walk with even step length, step timing and arm swing.

Common problems

If the pelite liner is difficult to don the number and thickness of the stump socks may be reduced. A nylon stump sock only may be used, but the physiotherapist must be extra vigilant about pressure areas. It is often necessary to vary the stump sock combination during treatment as the stump settles down during the early stages.

If the pelite fits but it is difficult to push into the hard socket, a nylon stump sock over the pelite will reduce the friction and should allow it to be pushed into the hard shell. (If a nylon sock is not available, try talcum powder, a plastic bag or the leg of a pair of tights.)

If the stump is grossly oedematous, it should be contained with either a bandage or Juzo sock (see Chapter 8) and elevated for about one hour before the prosthesis is tried. Alternatively, the patient could be mobilized on the pneumatic post-amputation mobility aid (Ppam Aid) prior to donning his prosthesis. If stump oedema persists, it may be due to poorly controlled congestive cardiac failure and a medical opinion should be sought.

If the socket is too loose the physiotherapist may increase the number of socks worn up to a total of three woollen socks. Any more than this alters the shape of the stump relative to the socket, but a woollen sock can be placed between the pelite and the hard socket if necessary. An appointment at the prosthetic centre should be made as this is an interim measure.

If the socket remains ill fitting and causes localized pressure problems or if the above remedies do not work, the physiotherapist must contact the Prosthetic Centre for an appointment. The prosthetist may line the pelite with leather, apply paratibial pads or try various other procedures to obtain a comfortable fit. If all the above procedures fail to make the limb comfortable, a new socket may be required (Barsby, 1989, personal communication).

Gait training

The new below-knee amputee will exercise initially in parallel bars with two hands and gradually reduce to one hand, and then to sticks. The following exercises should be included in his programme:

1. lateral weight transfer;
2. anterior–posterior weight transfer;
3. stepping forward for stance phase control;
4. swing the prosthesis forward for swing phase control;
5. stepping forward with the good leg (Karacoloff, 1985); and
6. hip hitching for the above-knee/below-knee prosthesis user.

As skin problems arise if the training is too vigorous, the prosthetic exercise sessions should be carefully timed by the therapist and increased in length as appropriate. If the wound is not healed or the stump is swollen, this must be closely monitored during gait training. As the patient progresses, walking is practised out of the parallel bars with suitable walking aid equipment. Before discharge, stairs, steps, slopes, outside uneven surfaces, transportation and getting up off the floor should be practised.

Common gait deviations

Excessive knee flexion

Characterized by:

1. excessive dorsiflexion of the foot or anterior tilt of the socket;
2. stiff plantaflexion bumper or heel cushion;
3. excessive anterior displacement of the socket over the foot; and
4. flexion contracture.

Insufficient knee flexion

Characterized by:

1. excessive plantaflexion of the foot;
2. soft plantaflexion bumper;
3. socket positioned posterior to the foot; and
4. weak quadriceps.

Excessive lateral thrust of the prosthesis

Characterized by:

1. excessive medial placement of the prosthetic foot; and
2. incorrect medio-lateral tilt of the socket.

Early knee flexion

Characterized by:

1. excessive anterior displacement of the socket over the foot;
2. excessive dorsiflexion of the foot;
3. excessive anterior tilt of the socket; and
4. soft dorsiflexion bumper.

Delayed knee flexion

Characterized by:

1. excessive post-displacement of the socket over the foot;
2. excessive plantaflexion of the foot;
3. excessive posterior tilt of the socket;
4. hard dorsiflexion bumper (University of Strathclyde, 1980b).

HIP DISARTICULATION PROSTHESES

In England and Wales in 1985 there were 50 new amputations around the hip referred for prostheses (Ham *et al.*, 1989). Due to this small

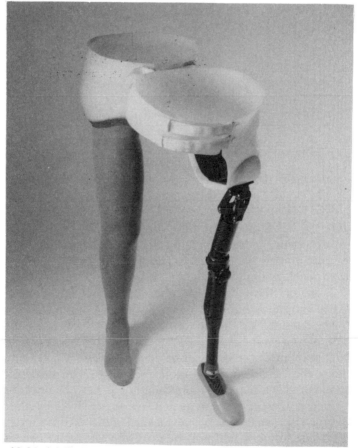

Figure 12.21 (a) Endolite modular hip disarticulation prosthesis.

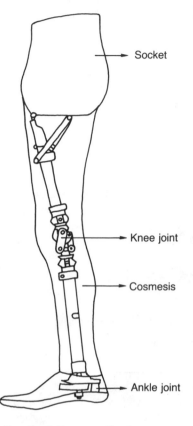

Figure 12.21 (b) Hip disarticulation prosthesis.

number, experience gained retaining these patients is limited. Experience tends to accumulate at centres, hospitals or DSCs that have large trauma or oncology units.

Until 1950, the through-hip amputee prosthesis was similar to the above-knee prosthesis but with more suspension and a saucer-shaped socket. The amputee sat on the hip joint as it was directly under him, giving an uneven sitting position (Waldes and Davis, 1979). In 1950, Colin McLaurin of Toronto developed a new design which is now used universally, the Canadian tilting table prosthesis. The suspension and stability required is achieved by enclosing the pelvis in a bucket-shaped socket (Figure 12.21a, b) and suspension is achieved by the socket shaping over the ischial crests. The socket is relieved anteriorly on the unaffected side to allow full movement of the hip joint. The socket is made of a rigid plastic laminate that is less rigid on the unaffected side to make it pliable for donning. The opening of the socket is generally at the anterior side and relief is given for the anterior and posterior iliac spines and the spinous processes of the vertebrae. The ischium rests on the cupped floor of the socket, which may be padded. The patient uses his pelvis and lumbar spine to move the leg forward and so a close fitting of the socket to the pelvis is essential. Although this design is an improvement on previous designs, the walking speed is limited, the gait is not aesthetic and the socket can be hot to wear (Sanders, 1986e). A four bar Endolite hip unit is now being used in the UK which gives a longer stride and better gait. It is 75% lighter than the older prosthesis as carbon fibre is used.

The floor of the Canadian socket should be level with the ground and the hip and knee joints have limiters on them to prevent hyperextension. The limb is set up 2.5 cm shorter than the opposite leg to help the patient clear the ground when walking. The prosthesis for the hemipelvectomy patient is similar to this but the bucket socket is modified and more complicated seating adaptations are required. There is little oedema, so casting takes place earlier than at some other levels.

Rehabilitation points

Donning

This prosthesis is generally found to be easiest to apply in standing with the leg propped up against the wall or corner of a room. It is important that the patient is well seated in the socket before it is securely fastened. No stump socks are available so patients are advised to wear cotton underwear with few seams or Seton's Tubigrip.

Check out

Close working with the prosthetist is important for these levels as the static and dynamic alignment of this limb are essential for its use (Waldes and Davis, 1979).

Use

This type of prosthesis can generally be worn for an hour at a time in the early rehabilitation phases, gradually increasing as the patient recovers. If the patient's sensation is reduced then it should be worn initially for less time (Karacoloff, 1985). A clear explanation of the amount of effort that is required to use such a prosthesis should be given early in the rehabilitation process.

Gait training

Patients should be taught to stand on their good side and hop with crutches as soon as possible following the operation. As they walk by tilting the pelvis this should be taught in both the lying and sitting positions.

The following gait exercises should be practised in parallel bars:

1. pelvic tilting;
2. swing through of the prosthesis; and
3. weight transference, moving the weight forward onto the prosthesis and eventually step through onto the good leg.

Once pelvic tilting and forward weight transference have been achieved, the full gait cycle training is continued. Equal step lengths, good rhythm and minimum deviation should be emphasized. Vaulting is commonly possible in the younger amputee who wants to walk faster.

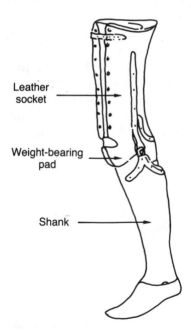

Leather socket

Weight-bearing pad

Shank

Figure 12.22 Knee disarticulation prosthesis (conventional).

208

KNEE DISARTICULATION OR THROUGH-KNEE PROSTHESES

Until recently, the knee disarticulation prosthesis was made of a contoured leather socket, which had a pad at the distal end for weight bearing and laced up anteriorly to provide suspension (Figure 12.22). There were two metal side steels, incorporating a higher knee joint attached to the socket and an exoskeletal shank.

Although this type of prosthesis is still available and used it is more common to see the knee disarticulation prosthesis that is a total contact,

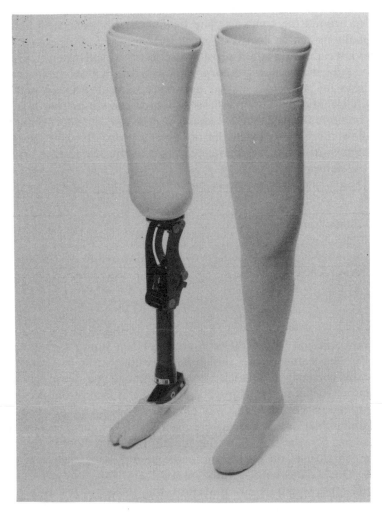

Figure 12.23 Knee disarticulation prosthesis (modern).

full weight-bearing socket which fits closely over the entire stump. It is made from a laminated plastic and to assist donning and doffing in one design an obturator window is cut into the socket medially to provide room for the femoral condyles to pass down the socket. The window position is held in place with velcro straps. Suspension is provided by the socket shape fitting closely around the femoral condyles (Figure 12.23). Alternatively the Miami design may be used in which an inner liner is made which follows the shape of the stump. The concave surfaces are fitted with a material which is compressed as the liner is inserted into the hard outer socket. Total contact and suspension are achieved by the close fit around the condyles. The loading in the socket can be taken proximally or distally by socket modification.

The knee disarticulation prosthesis functions well when a four bar linkage knee mechanism is incorporated which equalizes the level of the knee axes on both sides making gait more natural (Mensch and Ellis, 1987). Cosmetically, the prosthesis is poor in the sitting position as the thigh section is longer than the shank section and the short shank does not allow the foot to touch the floor. The prosthetic knee protrudes further towards than the unaffected leg and the knee centre is lower than the natural knee.

Rehabilitation points

Early weight bearing is practised by manual pressure on the stump in preparation for prosthetic use.

Donning

Whichever design of prosthesis is prescribed, a stump sock is applied initially. The leather socket design has an end-bearing pad which must be located correctly in the socket before donning. The stump is placed in the leather socket in the sitting position and it is laced from the bottom keeping the gap even all the way along the corset's length. If a pelvic band and ischial weight bearing are used, these are checked as with the above-knee prosthesis, as is the leg length. If a pelite liner is used this is applied in sitting and pushed onto the stump using the palm of the hands. Once the stump is fully inserted and the condyles correctly situated, the stump is inserted into the socket. This is generally performed in standing.

Check out

It is important to check that the end-bearing pad is in the correct position and that the end of the stump is correctly located in the pelite liner. The position of the adductor tendons and ischial tuberosity if an ischial platform is used should be checked as with the above-knee prosthesis. The leg length should be checked by using the therapist's hands over the iliac crests and the position of the anterior superior iliac spines. In sitting, the knee of the affected leg is longer than the natural knee due to either the knee mechanism or end-bearing pad.

Use

Ensure that the stump touches the endpad of the prosthesis. The amount of weight bearing that takes place is dependent on the type of amputation performed, for example Gritti-Stokes or through knee.

Common problems

If a leather socket is used the therapist must ensure that the corset is fastened evenly throughout its whole length for the correct fit and comfort. The amount of ischial weight bearing possible for each patient will depend on the type of amputation that has been performed.

Gait training

The knee disarticulation amputee develops an unnatural gait pattern as he has to stand in complete extension. In the stance phase these patients hold the hip in extension longer on the prosthetic leg compared with the good side (Mensch, 1983). Gait training follows the same principles as for the above-knee amputee but often a longer stride develops due to the longer remnant stump (Engstrom and Van de Ven, 1985).

SYME PROSTHESES

Syme amputations are more commonly seen in centres that deal with traumatic cases. The stump is similar to the through-knee stump in that it has a distal bulbous area. The standard Syme prosthesis was therefore similar to the through-knee prosthesis in that it had a leather socket or corset with laces which attached to the foot with side steels.

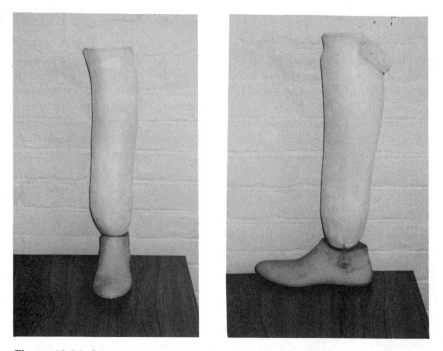

Figure 12.24 Syme prosthesis. (a) Anterior view, (b) side view.

In 1955 in Canada, a plastic Syme prosthesis was developed. The design incorporated a fixed anterior section and a posterior section that moved backwards like a door, to allow for donning. The 'door' was held in place by velcro straps. Today's Syme socket remains large compared with the amount of limb lost (Figure 12.24). The prosthesis incorporates a window to allow for donning and doffing within a total contact socket. The socket extends proximally to below the knee. An intimate socket fit is essential to ensure that weight bearing takes place on the heel pad correctly and that the pad does not move. It should also allow for calf muscle contraction. The window is generally placed on the medial aspect to maintain stump stability and is held closed with velcro straps.

In 1965 a more cosmetic elastic liner Syme prosthesis was developed in the USA. The liner (generally pelite) extends proximally until the diameter of bulbous end equals the calf diameter (Sanders, 1986f). The concave surface is fitted with a compressible foam which is pushed against the outer hard socket when donning occurs, ensuring a total contact socket and good suspension. Proximal weight bearing (i.e. a PTB or PTS) can be added to a Syme prosthesis and each patient is assessed individually to decide whether they will be proximally or distally weight bearing. There is a tendency for the heel pad in this amputation to move medially and posteriorly so stabilizing the heel pad prosthetically is very important (Fernie and Ruder, 1981a).

Rehabilitation points

Donning

As with the through-knee level, the type of prosthesis varies but the application is similar to that described in the through-knee section.

Check out

It is important to ensure that the end-bearing pad is correctly located and that it does not move with gait training. If proximal weight bearing is also used the correct location of the patella tendon bar should be checked.

Use

Training sessions should increase as the skin gradually hardens over the heel.

Common problems

If the position of the patient's own heel pad moves, discomfort and pain will be felt. Further surgery will be required to correct this.

Gait training

Balance activities and activities which incorporate push off should also be practised.

PARTIAL FOOT AMPUTATIONS

In the past a short leather ankle corset was attached to a wooden foot which was worn in a normal shoe. Today partial foot amputations (e.g. Chopart, Lisfranc) are generally fitted with shoe inserts and insoles. These can either be produced by the prosthetist or by an orthotist (shoe fitter). As the toe break action occurs between the remaining foot and the insert an ankle foot orthosis (splint) may be added for comfort.

Rehabilitation points

Care should be taken to see that the stump socks fit correctly and skin abrasions are avoided as these patients often have poor sensation. Exercises to maintain full range of movement at the remaining joints, balance work and push off exercises wearing the prosthesis should be practised.

OTHER CONSIDERATIONS

The bilateral amputee – the walker

The bilateral amputee will be assessed and treated according to the assessment findings. The medical condition, level of amputation, social and functional requirements will vary with each individual patient, as will their prosthetic prescription.

As discussed later in this chapter, the energy requirements for walking for the bilateral are much greater than for the normal subject and the presence of at least one knee joint increases the chance of the bilateral amputee becoming a successful prosthetic user. Bilateral Symes and below-knee amputees are therefore more likely to be successful walkers than bilateral above-knee amputees (Chapter 8).

Each prescription is individual and the timing of the amputations also influences the precription chosen. Amputees losing both legs together are generally dropped in height to assist gait training by lowering the centre of gravity. As the amputee becomes confident the length of the prostheses may be increased but generally the total height is kept below the amputee's original height. The bilateral above-knee amputee generally starts with rockers or stubbies without knee mechanisms and if successful they will both be increased in height and a knee mechanism will be added. The prostheses for the bilateral should emphasize ease of application, safety, comfort in wearing and use.

Functional activities

Once the amputee is confident and safe on his prosthesis, the exercise programme should include functional activities that are appropriate and

relevant to each individual's life-style. Full assessment by the physiotherapist and occupational therapist will ensure that all the areas are
covered practically. This will include activities from chairs, stairs,
slopes, uneven ground, picking up objects, kneeling, getting off the
floor and transportation (this is also covered in Chapter 8).

Alignment

Alignment of the components of the prosthesis in relation to each other
is done in two stages. Initially this is achieved at the work bench,
statically and then dynamically, when the amputee is wearing and
walking with the prosthesis, either by eyesight or gait analysis.

During walking, forces are acting downwards through the hip, knee
and ankle joints at different angles. These are called ground force
reaction vectors. Depending upon the position of this line of force, the
body's muscles will react to prevent the person falling over. If the vector
is too far over in one direction, a moment of force will develop and
cause excessive loading at one point of the prosthesis and incorrect
loading at another point.

When setting up a prosthesis the prosthetist uses these ground
reaction forces and aligns the socket in relation to the foot. In static
alignment the reference line is called the vertical reference line and runs
from the medial brim of the socket through the knee to the ankle. When
the knee position is being set, the trochanter, knee, ankle (TKA) line is
referred to (Fernie and Ruder, 1981a, b). The effect of the ground force
reaction vectors on gait deviations and their relevance to therapy are
discussed by other authors and are beyond the scope of this book
(Fernie and Ruder, 1981a, b; Sanders, 1986a; Mensch and Ellis, 1987).

Prosthetic socks

Socks are used with prostheses to provide an intimate fit, act as a
cushioning material, provide stability as the stump shrinks or swells, and
absorb sweat, therefore keeping the socket more hygienic. Socks should
be washed daily. There are three types of sock currently used: nylon,
cotton, towelling and wool and they come in different lengths and
widths. The thickness of the three types varies and this is used to
accommodate the alterations in stump volume. In the UK, one wool
sock is equal to the thickness of three cotton socks, for example. The
thinner socks can be used as cushioning next to the skin rather than wool

or used to help don and doff the prosthesis. Traditionally the wool socks were difficult to wash without shrinkage and matting occurring. Now new types of woollen socks are also becoming available that are easier to wash and maintain.

Activity legs

A variety of activity legs are available, for example swimming legs are available without joints for water activities. Active amputees in the UK should be encouraged to join the British Amputee Sports Association for advice on sport, participation in competitive games and national and international meetings.

Care of the prosthesis

The prosthesis should be stored carefully when not in use to prevent it falling over and cracking. The socket should be wiped daily with a damp cloth and its liner or insert removed from the socket and set aside to dry overnight. It is recommended that the endoskeletal models with foam cosmeses are stored flexed to help the foam to stretch (Karacoloff, 1985).

A Prescription Guide may be useful for the therapist working with amputees to ensure that no details of prosthetic prescription are overlooked (Rubin *et al.*, 1986).

Ambulation

Gait cycle

Normal gait is made up of two phases, swing and stance (Figure 12.18). During the stance phase, the heel comes into contact with the ground heel strike which is followed by the whole foot as the subject bears weight through that leg. Weight is then transmitted forwards onto the forefoot and lastly onto the big toe for the push off or toe off. Stance phase accounts for 60% of the gait cycle (Inman *et al.*, 1982). The swing phase begins at toe off and continues as the hip, knee and ankle are flexed and swung through in order to place the foot forwards at heel strike. The swing phase accounts for 40% of the gait cycle (Figure 12.25).

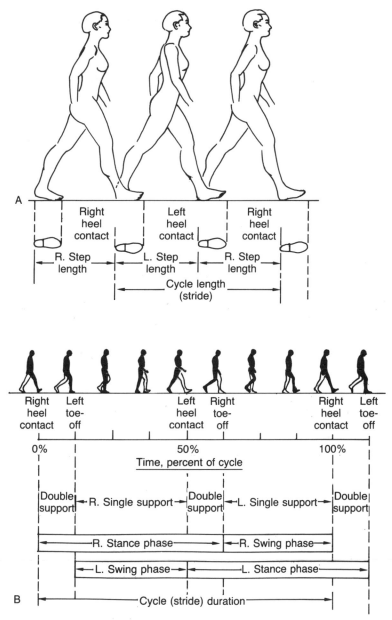

Figure 12.25 Distance and time dimensions of walking cycle. *A*, distance (length). *B*, time. From *Human Walking* by Inman, Ralston and Todd (1981), Williams and Wilkins, Baltimore.

During the gait cycle there is a period of double support when both feet are in contact with the ground at the same time. The length of time of this contact varies depending on the speed of walking. For example, when the subject is running there is no double support period. During the walking cycle, the pelvis drops approximately 5 cm between the mid stance and double support phases – vertical displacement. The centre of gravity is displaced laterally approximately 5 cm, as weight is transferred from leg to leg – lateral displacement (Inman et al., 1982). The width of the walking base is usually between 5 and 10 cm in the adult. The number of steps taken by the subject per minute is called *cadence* and varies from between 70 and 130 steps per minute, depending on the subject's walking speed. During walking the hip angle changes from 25° of flexion through to 25° of extension. The knee angle varies from 0° to 60° in the toe off phase. The ankle angle varies from 15° dorsiflexion to 20° in plantaflexion.

Amputees walk more slowly than normal people in an effort to keep their percentage of energy utilization close to normal and to maintain heart rate and cardiac output at a constant (English, 1981). Non-vascular amputees do not adjust their speed as much as vascular subjects. Traumatic amputees were found to walk at the following speeds: below knee, 71 m/min; through knee, 61 m/min and above knee, 52 m/min. The vascular below-knee amputees walked at 45 m/min and above-knee amputees at 36 m/min. All amputee groups, except the vascular above-knee group, walked with less effort using a prosthesis (Sulzle et al., 1978). Below-knee amputees walk generally faster than above-knee patients and even at equal speeds they require less energy. Their work capacity has been found to increase with endurance training and general strengthening exercises. Oxygen consumption has been found to be 9% higher than the normal in a single below-knee amputee, 49% higher in a single above-knee amputee and 280% higher in a bilateral above-knee amputee (Chi-Tsou et al., 1979).

It has also been found that a patient with a short below-knee stump (<6% of total body height) requires more energy to walk (40%) than a patient with a longer stump (Gonzalez et al., 1974) (i.e. >8% total body height). Renström (1981) found that the walking speed of subjects increased from 34 m/min at the start of training to 53 m/min after training (this was 64% of the normal speed of a healthy subject). The gait velocity for vascular amputees was 66% at Syme levels, 59% at below-knee level and 44% of the normal at above-knee level. For the traumatic amputees these figures were 87% for the below-knee amputee and 63% for the above-knee amputee (Waters et al., 1976).

The more joints and muscles that are lost and replaced by a

prosthesis, the greater the loss of the normal locomotor mechanism and therefore the greater the energy cost of ambulation as well as the degree of disability (Fisher and Gullickson, 1978). Walking with a locked knee produces a higher walking velocity with lower effort and is therefore suitable for the older patient. In the younger above-knee amputee, using a free knee produces greater energy expenditure and heart rate but the physical condition of the younger patient is able to cope with this (Isakov *et al.*, 1985).

Many patients over 65 years of age require nearly a year to achieve their maximum walking potential (Kerstein *et al.*, 1975). Their sensory input is decreased as well as their tactile, visual olfactory and auditory systems. Often there is also visual loss. The elderly are slow to learn and less able to absorb new ideas. They have reduced short-term memory and find new tasks difficult to learn. Their strength, endurance, agility and reduction time are reduced and they are generally less active with multiple diseases.

Amputees should be able to walk more than 600 steps a day in order to function at a minimal level of activity with a moderate amount of support in a single storey house. If there is no support at home, this should be increased to 1100 steps a day and a two storey dwelling would increase these figures by 25%. In another study, Holden and Fernie (1987) found that the elderly and above-knee amputees could not do this at discharge and the number of steps they could take reduced as time from discharge increased (Holden and Fernie, 1987; *et al.*, 1987). In a recent study of above-knee amputees most patients were found to achieve their maximum before discharge (Beckman and Axtell, 1987).

In these times of dwindling resources it is important to look closely at prosthetic use. The patient's attitude is the most important factor in prosthetic use. Those who have the determination to walk will do so in any situation (Weaver and Marshall, 1973). A below-knee amputee is more likely to use a prosthesis than an above-knee amputee. Bilateral amputees are less likely to be users than single amputees of the same level. Bilateral below-knee amputees are more likely to use prostheses than an above-knee amputee. Wheelchair propulsion has been found to be a more energy-efficient mode of mobility for the elderly bilateral amputee than ambulation (DuBow *et al.*, 1983). Good range of movement, strength and compliance with prosthetic fitting and training are positive criteria for successful prosthetic use (Mueller and Delitto, 1985). Ninety per cent of the population are right-hand dominant and it has been found that right-sided amputees take longer to rehabilitate (Kerstein *et al.*, 1977).

REFERENCES

Beckman, C.E. and Axtell, L.A. (1987) Prosthetic use in elderly patients with dysvascular above knee and through knee amputations. *Phys. Ther.*, **67**, 1510–1516.

Beswick, J.B. (1986) Evaluation of the Seattle foot. *J. Rehab. Res. Dev.*, **23**, 77–94.

Chi-Tsou, H., Jackson, J.R. and Moore, N.B. (1979) Amputation: energy cost of ambulation. *Arch. Phys. Med. Rehabil.*, **60**, 18–24.

DuBow, L.L., Witt, P.L., Kadaba, M.P., Reyes, R. and Cochran, G.V.B. (1983) Oxygen consumption of elderly persons with bilateral below knee amputations: Ambulation vs. wheelchair propulsion. *Arch. Phys. Med. Rehabil.*, **64**, 255–259.

Edelstein, J.E. (1988) Prosthetic feet; state of the art. *Phys. Ther.*, **68**, 1874–1881.

English, A.W.G. and Dean, A.A.G. (1980) The artificial limb service. *Health Trends*, **12**, 77–82.

English, E. (1981) The energy costs of walking for the Lower Extremity Amputee, in *Amputation Surgery and Rehabilitation: the Toronto Experience* (ed. J.P. Kostuik), Churchill Livingstone, Edinburgh, pp. 311–314.

Engstrom, B. and Van de Ven, C. (1985) The through knee levels of amputation, in *Physiotherapy for Amputees. The Roehampton Approach*, Churchill Livingstone, Edinburgh, pp. 138–147.

Fernie, G.R. and Ruder, K. (1981a) Lower limb prosthetics, in *Amputation Surgery and Rehabilitation: the Toronto Experience* (ed. J.P. Kostuik), Churchill Livingstone, Edinburgh, pp. 267–291.

Fernie, G.R. and Ruder, K. (1981b) Biomechanics of gait and prosthetic alignment, in *Amputation Surgery and Rehabilitation: the Toronto Experience* (ed. J.P. Kostuik), Churchill Livingstone, Edinburgh, pp. 267–291.

Fisher, S.V. and Gullickson, G. (1978) Energy cost of ambulation in health and disability. A literature review. *Arch. Phys. Med. Rehabil.*, **59**, 124–133.

Fishman, S., Edelstein, J.E. and Krebs, D.E. (1987) Icelandic Swedish New York above knee prosthetic sockets: paediatric experience. *J. Paed. Orthop.*, **7**, 557–562.

Flandry, F., Beskin, J., Chambers, R.B., Perry, J., Waters, R.L. and Chauez, R. (1989) The effect on the CAT – CAM above knee prosthesis on functional rehabilitation. *Clin. Orthop. Rel. Res.*, **239**, 249–262.

Goh, J.C.H., Solomonidis, S.E., Spence, W.D. and Paul, J.P. (1984) Biomechanical evaluation of SACH and uniaxial feet. *Prosthet. Orthot. Int.*, **8**, 147–154.

Gonzalez, E.G., Corcoran, P.J. and Reyes, R.L. (1974) Energy expenditure in below knee amputees; correlation with stump length. *Arch. Phys. Med. Rehabil.*, **55**, 111–119.

Ham, R.O., Roberts, V.C. and Luff, R. (1989) A five-year review of referrals for prosthetic treatment in England, Wales and Northern Ireland, 1981–85. *Health Trends*, **21**, 2–5.

Holden, J.M. and Fernie, G.R. (1983) Minimal walking levels for amputees living at home. *Physiotherapy Canada*, **35**, 317–320.

Holden, J.M. and Fernie, G.R. (1987) Extent of artificial limb use following rehabilitation. *J. Orthopaed. Res.*, **5**, 562–568.

Inman, V.T., Ralston, H.J. and Todd, F. (1981) *Human walking*. Williams and Wilkins.

Isakov, E., Susak, Z. and Becker, E. (1985) Energy expenditure and cardiac response in above knee amputees while using prostheses with open and locked knee mechanisms. *Scand. J. Rehab. Med.*, Suppl. **12**, 108–111.

Karacoloff, L.A. (1985) Prosthetic training, in *Lower Extremity Amputation: a Guide to Functional Outcomes in Physical Therapy Management*, pp. 65–82. Aspen Publication, Rockville, Maryland.

Kerstein, M.D., Zimmer, H., Dungdale, F.E. and Lerner, E. (1975) What influence does age have on rehabilitation of amputees. *Geriatrics*, December, **39**, 67–71.

Kerstein, M.D., Zimmer, H., Dugdale, F.E. and Lerner, E. (1977) Successful rehabilitation following amputation of dominant versus non dominant extremities. *Am. J. Occup. Ther.*, **31**, 313–315.

Mensch, G. (1983) Physiotherapy following through knee amputation. *Prosthet. Orthot. Int.*, **7**, 79–87.

Mensch, G. (1984) ISPO seminar features new flexible socket for amputees. *Physiotherapy Canada*, **36**, 208–209.

Mensch, G. and Ellis, P.M. (1987) Prosthetics and prosthetic gait, in *Physical Therapy Management of Lower Extremity Amputations*, Heinemann Physiotherapy, London, pp. 201–335.

Mueller, M.J. and Delitto, A. (1985) Selective criteria for successful long-term prosthetic use. *Phys. Ther.*, **65**, 1037–1040.

Öberg, K.E.T. and Kamwendo, K. (1988) Knee components for the above knee amputation, in *Amputation Surgery and Lower Limb Prosthetics*, Blackwell Scientific, Oxford, pp. 152–171.

Picken, R.R. (1985) The above knee prosthesis, in *Lower Extremity Amputation: a Guide to Functional Outcomes in Physical Therapy Management*, pp. 31–36. Aspen Publication, Rockville, Maryland.

Radcliffe, C.W. (1977) Above knee prosthesis. *Prosthet. Orthot. Int.*, **1**, 146–160.

Renström, P. (1981) Below knee amputees at an Amputee Training Centre, in *The Below-knee Amputee*, University of Göteborg, Sweden, pp. 31–44.

Roberts, R.A. (1986) Suction socket suspension for below knee amputees. *Arch. Phys. Med. Rehabil.*, **67**, 196–199.

Rubin, G., Fischer, E. and Dixon, M. (1986) Prescription of above-knee and below-knee prostheses. *Prosthet. Orthot. Int.*, **10**, 117–124.

Sanders, G.T. (1986a) Statistics, in *Lower Limb Amputation: a Guide to Rehabilitation*, F.A. Davis Co., Philadelphia, pp. 35–55, (b) Above knee, pp. 231–254, (c) Knee mechanisms, pp. 258–274, (d) Ankle/foot mechanisms, pp. 143–160, (e) Below knee, pp. 163–204, (f) Hip disarticulations, pp. 277–294, (g) Ankle disarticulation and Syme, pp. 121–140.

Staats, T.B. and Lundir, J. (1987) The UCLA total surface bearing suction below knee prosthesis. *Clin. Pros. and Orthotics*, **11**, (3), 118–130.

Sulzle, H., Pagliarulo, M., Rodgers, M. and Jordan, C. (1978) Energetics of amputee gait. *Orthop. Clin. North Am.*, **9**. 358–362.

University of Strathclyde (1980a) Above knee gait analysis, in *Lower Limb Prosthetics*, National Centre for Training and Education in Prosthetics and Orthotics, Glasgow.

University of Strathclyde (1980b) Below knee gait analysis and deviations, in

Lower Limb Prosthetics, National Centre for Training and Education in Prosthetics and Orthotics, Glasgow.

Waldes, J.D. and Davis, B.C. (1979) Prosthetic sitting and points of rehabilitation for hindquarter and hip disarticulation patients. *Physiotherapy*, **65**, 4–6.

Waters, R.L., Perry, J., Antonelli, D. and Hislop, H. (1976) Energy cost of walking of amputees: the influence of level of amputation. *J. Bone Joint Surg.*, **58**, 42–46.

Weaver, P.C. and Marshall, S.A. (1973) A functional and social review of lower limb amputees. *Br. J. Surg.*, **60**, 732–737.

APPENDIX 12.1: COMMON PROSTHETIC TERMS

No. 1 Standard	For hip disarticulation or hemipelvectomy.
Canadian tilting table	As above but with adjustable hip limiter and modular hip joint.
No. 2	For above knee with rigid pelvic band or double swivel pelvic band (i.e. hip joint).
No. 3	For above knee with soft suspension, i.e. shaped leather belt, roller cords or elastic, silesian belt or self-suspending, i.e. Suction, TSC, TSB.
No. 6	For through knee shaped over condyles for self-suspension usually end bearing or with pelvic band or waist belt.
No. 7	For below knee with very short stumps or flexion contracture. Suspension as for No. 6 fitted as kneeling limb.
No. 8	For below knee with thigh corset. With various suspensions, e.g. waist belt, shoulder strap, cross knee strap.
No. 12	For below knee with or without patella tendon bearing, cuff or elastic stocking suspension. Light metal exoskeletal.
PTB	For below knee, patella tendon bearing, suspension as for No. 12. Endoskeletal, can be self-suspending, e.g. PTS.
No. 13	For Symes with side steels 'enclosed' – for Symes as No. 12 self-suspension or gaiter suspension.
No. 16	For Symes with weight-bearing thigh corset.
RPB	Rigid pelvic band.
DSPB	Double swivel pelvic band.
TES	Total elastic suspension.

MAP	Modular assembly prosthesis.
SAKL	Semi automatic knee lock.
EBA	Extension bias aids (pick ups).
HOKL	Hand operated knee lock.
WTKL	Wheel type knee control.
ICS	Internal coil spring or internal calf spring.
BSK	Blatchford stabilizing knee.
ESK	Endolite stabilized knee.
SPC	Swing phase control: pneumatic, hydraulic, variable vane, e.g. PSPC.
PTB	Patella tendon bearing.
SACH	Solid ankle cushion heel.
MUF	Moulded uniaxial foot.
PFR	Pylon forefoot rocker.
SRP	Short rocker pylons.
TSC	Total surface contact.
TSB	Total surface bearing.
PTS	Patella tendon supracondylar/suprapatella.
CAT/CAM	Contoured adducted trochanteric/controlled alignment method.
NSNA	Natural shape natural alignment socket.
ISNY	Iceland, Sweden, New York socket.

Index